Strategic Public Diplomacy

AND

American Foreign Policy

Strategic Public Diplomacy

AND

American Foreign Policy

The Evolution of Influence

JAROL B. MANHEIM

New York   *Oxford*

OXFORD UNIVERSITY PRESS

1994

Oxford University Press

Oxford   New York   Toronto
Delhi   Bombay   Calcutta   Madras   Karachi
Kuala Lumpur   Singapore   Hong Kong   Tokyo
Nairobi   Dar es Salaam   Cape Town
Melbourne   Auckland   Madrid

and associated companies in
Berlin   Ibadan

Copyright © 1994 by Jarol B. Manheim

Library of Congress Cataloging-in-Publication Data
Manheim, Jarol B., 1946–
Strategic public diplomacy and American Foreign Policy :
the evolution of influence / Jarol B. Manheim.
p. cm.   Includes bibliographical references and index.
ISBN 0–19–508737–2
ISBN 0–19–508738–0 (pbk.)
1. United States—Foreign relations—1945– —Case studies.
2. International relations—Psychological aspects.
3. Public relations and politics.
4. Lobbying.   5. Foreign agents. I. Title.
JX1417.M326   1993   327'.01'9—dc20   93–40827

Portions of this book are based on work previously published or in press, and are adapted or reproduced here with permission. These include parts of Chapter 4 drawn from Jarol B. Manheim, ''The War of Images: Strategic Communication in the Gulf Conflict,'' in Stanley A. Renshon, ed., *The Political Psychology of the Gulf War: Leaders, Publics, and the Process of Conflict* (Pittsburgh: University of Pittsburgh Press, 1993), and from Jarol B. Manheim, ''Strategic Public Diplomacy: Managing Kuwait's Image During the Gulf Conflict,'' in W. Lance Bennett and David Paletz, eds., *Taken By Storm: The Media, Public Opinion, and Foreign Policy in the Gulf War* (Chicago: University of Chicago Press, in press); Chapter 6 from Jarol B. Manheim, ''Rites of Passage: The 1988 Seoul Olympics as Public Diplomacy,'' *Political Research Quarterly* 43 (1990): pp. 279–295 (reprinted by permission of the University of Utah, copyright holder); Chapter 7 from Jarol B. Manheim and Robert B. Albritton, ''Insurgent Violence versus Image Management: The Struggle for National Images in Southern Africa,'' *British Journal of Political Science* 17 (1987): pp. 201–218, and ''Changing National Images: International Public Relations and Media Agenda Setting,'' *American Political Science Review* 78 (1984): 641–654; and Chapter 8 from Jarol B. Manheim, ''A Model of Agenda Dynamics,'' in Margaret L. McLaughlin, ed., *Communication Yearbook 10* (Beverly Hills: Sage, 1987).

1 3 5 7 9 8 6 4 2

Printed in the United States of America
on acid-free paper

For Amy and Laura

Preface

The research reported in this volume is the product of some fifteen years of effort. It began innocently enough shortly after New Years Day in 1979 when I sat down with a copy of the *Wall Street Journal* to read over lunch. The front page—actually, the left-hand column, as I recall—carried a piece under the headline "Public Relations Firms Draw Fire for Aiding Repressive Countries." The story described several such efforts.

The difference between journalism and social science is that the journalist is more taken with description, and the social scientist with assessment and explanation. So it was that, though the story greatly piqued my interest, it did not satisfy my curiosity. I began to wonder whether such efforts as those described by the newspaper actually had any effect on public opinion or governmental policy. Together with a colleague, Robert Albritton, I decided to find out. The observations and analyses you find here are the product of the odyssey that followed. As is so often the case, a simple question did not have a simple answer.

Though I have found this subject personally fascinating, it is not only my interest in the strategic representation of foreign interests in the United States that has grown over the intervening decade and a half. As the evidence in this volume will show, during this same period, the very practice of this art-cum-science of influence has expanded as well—not only in scale, but in the degree of sophistication brought to the task by those who deliver U.S.-directed media, public, and government affairs management services to foreign governments and corporations. International strategic communication has been one of the leading growth industries of the 1980s and 1990s—a true American success story.

In one sense, this is not a new phenomenon. For many years now, foreign interests have sought representation in Washington, often in the form of professional lobbyists whose influence and access they hoped to rent and use to advantage. But in another, it is quite new. For what we see now are increasingly comprehensive efforts—often focusing on grass-roots organizing and systematic media management—that look very little like the canyons of Gucci loafers and the smoke-filled rooms that accord with the commonplace public image of special interest representation. Rather, they resemble nothing so much as political campaigns. And that is precisely what they are—political campaigns whose objective is not the election of a candidate to office, but the advancement of some policy of interest to the client government or corporation.

The reason for this change is quite straightforward. The lobbyists who have long dominated the representation of foreign interests are gradually but steadily being replaced by individuals and firms with experience in managing domestic political campaigns. And these relative newcomers are simply doing what they know best. But they are doing it for clients who pay much more money than do most political candidates and whose business is substantially less cyclical. What we have in place, then, is a transformation in the mix of skills that are applied to foreign agentry, reinforced by a compelling set of economic incentives, not the least of which is to eat and find shelter during odd-numbered years. It is the purpose of this book to explore both of these dynamics—the intellectual and the economic—as they affect the representation of foreign interests in the United States and its impact on the making of U.S. foreign policy.

Because the emphasis here is on the contemporary practice of interest representation, we will focus a good deal more attention on the public relations aspects of public diplomacy, and rather less on traditional lobbying. In the end, the two cannot be disaggregated one from the other, and many of the examples discussed in these pages had both public relations and lobbying components. But it is my judgment that political management is displacing over-the-desk lobbying in both scale and influence. That judgment has guided the selection and organization of the material presented here.

Though this is not a subject that generally tops the public's political agenda, it has emerged from obscurity in recent years. Writers like Pat Choate and organizations like the Center for Public Integrity have called attention to what they perceive as the evils inherent in foreign agentry, and H. Ross Perot has made elimination of the practices described here into a cornerstone of his program of political reform. What unites these and other polemics on the topic is their clear intent to discredit the representation of foreign interests by American consultants.

Those who anticipate yet another such effort here are destined for disappointment. For my purpose in this volume is not to decry the practice of international strategic public diplomacy, but to illuminate it so that, as the contemporary debate over this important issue develops, it can be based to some extent on fact—on the nature, extent, and probable influence of these propaganda-like activities—and to some extent on reasoned and analytical judgments about the phenomenon in question, rather than on pejorative rhetoric. There are real issues here, and our judgments about them ought to be informed and rational, an outcome to which I hope to contribute.

I owe an immeasurable debt of gratitude to Bob Albritton, without whose interest in the subject, and whose unequalled command of interrupted time-series analysis, this project would never have gotten off the ground. Thanks, Bob. And thanks, too, to Susan Helgeth, Bob Jones, and David Reed, whose coding and other efforts over the years made the early stages of this research possible. Thanks to Lee Jong Ryool and Yoon Ki Byung, for facilitating my access to ranking journalists and government officials in the Republic of Korea, and to the Korea Press Center, the International Cultural Society of Korea, and the Office of the Press Secretary to the President of the Republic of Korea for their support of portions of the research. Thanks to everyone in the various governments and consulting firms who took the time to speak with me about their experiences—and especially to those who were candid. Thanks to the late Morris Davis for sharing his insights; to Dave Paletz for his valued critiques of more than one piece of this opus at various professional meetings; to Steven Livingston, whose comments on an early draft offered a valuable guide to revision, and to others who have similarly and collectively been of great assistance; and to Dina Zinnes, for yielding to persuasion and logic at a critical moment. Thanks to David Roll, my editor at Oxford, whose comments and suggestions were almost invariably incisive and directly on target . . . and who knew when to give in. Thanks to Ellie Fuchs of the Oxford staff and Catherine Clements, who copy edited the manuscript. And special thanks to Dick Merritt, who somehow saw the merit of this enterprise early on, even through the haze of early drafts of early papers, and helped more than once to steer it through the whitewater.

For all of the guidance and assistance I have received from these and other folks over the years, I remain as stubborn as ever. So the errors and failures of insight that you might find in reading this book are undoubtedly mine. In discovering them, I hope that you, too, will help to advance the debate.

Washington, D.C.   J. B. M.
October 1993

Contents

I Strategic Public Diplomacy

II Case Studies in Strategic Public Diplomacy

III Analysis and Implications

I

Strategic Public Diplomacy

Diplomacy is to do and say
The nastiest thing in the nicest way
Isaac Goldberg, *The Reflex*

1

Propaganda in the Age of Strategic Communication

Nations have long recognized the importance of managing the perceptions of them that governments and citizens of other countries hold. The Italian spin doctor, Niccolo Machiavelli, in his treatise *The Prince,* is often credited as the progenitor of strategic political communication, but, in truth, the phenomenon predates him. When Richard I of England during the Crusades ordered the eyes plucked from hundreds of prisoners and sent to his rival, Saladin, and when Vlad the Impaler (whose deeds gave rise to the Dracula legend) ordered the decapitation of some ten thousand of his most loyal subjects and the literal posting of their heads around the borders of his kingdom, each was sending across the equivalent of national boundaries a message of unmistakable clarity. Diplomatic practice has generally mellowed a bit in more recent times, but a recognition of the need of governments to communicate with the leaders and peoples of other lands endures.

Though the centrality of communication to the conduct of diplomacy has long been evident, both scholars and practitioners have devoted more systematic attention to this relationship in recent years than previously. This renewed emphasis can be characterized as addressing four distinctive aspects of diplomatic activity: government-to-government, diplomat-to-diplomat, people-to-people, and government-to-people contacts.

The first of these refers to the traditional form of diplomacy, the exchange of formal messages between sovereign states. The new em-

3

phasis here is typified by Raymond Cohen (1987), who explores the nuances of form in diplomatic exchanges with particular attention to the rituals and cues that accompany and give added meaning to the various communiques.

The second, commonly termed "personal diplomacy," refers to the individual-level interactions among those involved in diplomatic contacts. The value ascribed to personal diplomacy is often cited at an institutional level as a rationale for summitry (e.g., for the seemingly routinized meetings of American and Russian leaders or of the leaders of the principal Western economies) and has been addressed as a subject of scholarly inquiry by Harold Saunders (1988), who ascribes particular importance to the interpersonal relationships among diplomats themselves.

The third, often referred to as "public diplomacy," is characterized by cultural exchanges such as the Fulbright Program, media development initiatives, and the like, all designed to explain and defend government policies and portray a nation to foreign audiences.

The last, which is another form of public diplomacy, identified by W. Philips Davison (1974) and Richard L. Merritt (1980), includes efforts by the government of one nation to influence public or elite opinion in a second nation for the purpose of turning the foreign policy of the target nation to advantage. It is this latter aspect of diplomatic activity that provides the context for the present analysis.

In its earliest incarnation, the twentieth-century study of what was then commonly referred to as "propaganda" was extensive indeed. The research of Carl Hovland, Harold Lasswell, Wilbur Schramm, Morris Janowitz, Irving Janis, and others, received substantial government support, especially following the outbreak of World War II, and gave impetus to the development of social psychology and to early interest in political communication.[1] In the United States, propaganda was at once an accepted instrument of government—as exemplified by George Creel and the Committee on Public Information—and an object of fear to be investigated by the House Committee on Un-American Activities, depending, in large measure, on the direction of informational flow (Lee, 1952).

The study of propaganda during this period took two principal tracks, one, as noted, directed at the psychological mechanics of influence, and the second at the specific techniques by which propagandists ostensibly plied their trade. The first of these tracks led scholars to a more general and largely empirical examination of attitudes and such attitude-related processes as change or inoculation against change. The second led to an interest in political public relations, advertising, and marketing which tends to be expressed in more anecdotal and generally more normative terms. A review of scholarship on propaganda from this period lies beyond the scope of this volume, but it is important to note that both approaches have had enduring influence in such disciplines as communication, political science, and psychology.

More recently, the term "public diplomacy" has come into vogue to characterize activities that would once have been described as propaganda. According to Gifford D. Malone (1988: 12), the term was reportedly coined in 1965 by Edmund Gullion of the Fletcher School of Law and Diplomacy at Tufts University. It has been defined as "a government's process of communicating with foreign publics in an attempt to bring about understanding for its nation's ideas and ideals, its institutions and culture, as well as its national goals and current policies" (Tuch, 1990). Thus, the Voice of America (VOA) (and the international broadcast services of other countries), created in 1942 to counteract the presumed effects abroad of Nazi wartime propaganda broadcasts, now engages in "public diplomacy," as do the libraries maintained overseas by the United States Information Service, the participants in the Fulbright exchange program, and other persons and agencies. In no small measure, this change in label represents a lesson learned from the propagandists themselves—that what one calls an object helps to determine how it is perceived by others. But in part, it also represents a sort of gentrification of the art of influence reflective of the greater legitimacy that attends to such functions in a world more accustomed to bombardment by mediated messages.

Public diplomacy is both public and diplomatic. International broadcasters, for example, maintain regular schedules that are widely publicized through such means as the annual *World Radio and TV Handbook* and encourage audience participation through special mailings, contests, and the like, all of which are conducted in plain view and with the full knowledge of any target government that might be interested. The messages do, in some instances, reflect overt or subtle points of view, but the technique generally eschews the sort of fear- and hate-mongering of an earlier era (Abshire, 1976; Deibel and Roberts, 1976). As John Lee put it in the preface to his book, *The Diplomatic Persuaders* (1968),

It is no longer possible for high-level statesmen to glide through the
lofty avenues of diplomacy, trailed by first, second, and third secretaries in perfect protocol alignment. A government, to survive, must
supplement formal government-to-government relations with an approach to the people. . . . To meet this challenge governments
around the world have turned to a totally new concept of international
diplomacy. This is the age of public diplomacy. . . . International
opinion wields incredible power, and we must inform the people of
other nations . . . , allies and enemies alike. The government that
fails to do so may find itself inarticulate in the face of world opinion.
(pp. ix–x)

On two occasions, Congress has held hearings to examine the organization, conduct, and effectiveness of U.S. efforts at public diplomacy (United States House of Representatives, 1977, 1987). The general
conclusion has been that such activities could productively be expanded
and improved. In the present context, however, the most revealing
governmental inquiry might be that conducted in the late 1970s by
the U.S. General Accounting Office (GAO). In a 1979 report (United
States General Accounting Office, 1979), the GAO summarized the
public diplomacy activities of seven countries—France, Great Britain, Japan, West Germany, China, and the Soviet Union, as well as
the United States—and assessed their implications for U.S. foreign
policy. After noting that public diplomacy has become a major instrument of foreign policy for the United States and other nations and
describing the U.S. effort as smaller than those of both allies and adver-
saries, the GAO offered six avenues for improvement: greater cooperation with public diplomacy efforts of U.S. allies to improve efficiency,
improved financial management, expanded emphasis on the teaching of
English (e.g., through VOA broadcasts), limited legalization of the
domestic distribution of U.S. Information Agency (USIA) produced
materials,[2] adequate compensation of overseas public diplomacy representatives, and a more systematic assessment of Soviet public diplomacy in the United States. Leaving aside the "bean counter" mentality
that seems to characterize these recommendations, they do reflect as
well the general approach of the U.S. government to public diplomacy
during this period, which was grounded in a belief that relatively
straightforward efforts to disseminate information that accorded with the
U.S. viewpoint to the largest possible audience in the greatest number of
countries, while keeping a bit of a wary eye on those targeting their

efforts in the other direction, would best serve the interests of the United States. Scholarship enlightened by this perspective has tended to focus on issues relating to the management, general content and direction, and integration with larger foreign policy interests and initiatives, of public diplomacy efforts (e.g., Green, 1988; Malone, 1988; Smith, 1980; Tuch, 1990).[3]

The most contemporary approach to this set of phenomena, and the one that will frame the balance of this book, is perhaps best described as an emphasis on *"strategic* public diplomacy." Strategic public diplomacy is the international manifestation of a relatively new style of information management that I have characterized elsewhere (1991a), drawing on use of the term by some practitioners, as "strategic political communication." In this view, political communication encompasses the creation, distribution, control, use, processing, and effects of information as a political resource, whether by governments, organizations, groups, or individuals. *Strategic* political communication incorporates the use of sophisticated knowledge of such attributes of human behavior as attitude and preference structures, cultural tendencies, and media-use patterns—as well as knowledge of such relevant organizational behaviors as how news organizations make decisions regarding news content and how congressional committees schedule and structure hearings—to shape and target messages so as to maximize their desired impact while minimizing undesired collateral effects. Strategic public diplomacy, then, is public diplomacy practiced less as an art than as an applied transnational science of human behavior. It is, within the limits of available knowledge, the practice of propaganda in the earliest sense of the term, but enlightened by half a century of empirical research into human motivation and behavior.[4]

As early as 1966, scholars and practitioners had begun to recognize the potential for developing a more sophisticated approach to the conduct of public diplomacy. In that year, the Bernays Foundation (named for Edward L. Bernays, commonly regarded as the father of modern public relations practice) sponsored a series of lectures on the topic at Tufts University. Later published in an anthology (Hoffman, 1968), these essays covered the applicability of such bodies of knowledge as public opinion research, national cultures, group dynamics, psychological operations, and semantics and linguistics to the problem at hand. Participants included Lloyd Free, Margaret Mead, Lewis Coser, and Daniel Lerner, to name but a few.

Subsequently, Fisher (1972) outlined in a rather more orderly fashion the social scientific knowledge base on which increasingly sophisticated efforts at public diplomacy might be grounded. He argued that expanding communications technologies and greater public participation in foreign affairs policymaking were challenging the traditional means of conducting international relations in ways that must be taken into account. Davis (1977), in a case study of Nigerian politics surrounding the period of that country's civil war, pointed to the significance of public relations and other consultants in representing the political interests of governments and various subnational organizations to external audiences, notably in the United States and other Western industrialized countries. These efforts, he found, were of value not only in framing images held by the audiences of the various foreign clients, but in translating those images into relatively advantageous policy outcomes. And a few years later, Merritt (1980) suggested that governments had indeed developed a greater appreciation for the role of information campaigns as instruments of their respective foreign policies, and for the more or less subtle techniques available to them to implement such efforts. Robert Albritton and I were able to document the effectiveness of these campaigns, and some of their limitations, in a series of studies that identified and tested a particular model of image change in which the goals of image management were shown to vary depending on certain key characteristics of the initial media portrayal of the country in question (Manheim and Albritton, 1984, 1986, 1987; Albritton and Manheim, 1983, 1985; Manheim, 1987).

More recently, Anderson (1989) has offered a case study of the Reagan administration's marshaling of the tools of strategic public diplomacy to influence U.S. media and public perceptions of Nicaragua and the Sandinistas, Choate (1990) has presented an extensive examination of the representation of Japanese governmental and corporate interests in the domestic political arena of the United States, and the Center for Public Integrity (1993) has documented the elaborate public relations campaign employed by Mexico in its pursuit of congressional approval of the North American Free Trade Agreement. Choate, in particular, has demonstrated the intertwining of political and commercial interests, in effect, the partnership of government and business, in the design and conduct of public diplomacy, at least by some countries. Finally, Fisher (1987: 134–35), not surprisingly given his earlier contribution, has called for a more pro-active role for the USIA in U.S. foreign policymaking, first by fostering more systematically the psychological infrastructure that would sustain a more sophisticated U.S. effort, and second by bringing its expertise in communication and in psychology to bear in the formative stages of the policy process rather than in implementation alone. There is some evidence that Fisher's call has been heeded, if not by the State Department, at least by the Department of Defense (Kriesel, 1985).

From these studies and related literature, when considered in the aggregate, we know that:

- There exists a knowledge base in such disciplines as communication, journalism, political science, and psychology sufficient to guide relatively sophisticated efforts at strategic communication, which efforts can be employed to further the interests of governments in the international system.
- Such strategic approaches to public diplomacy, grounded in social scientific knowledge regarding attitude structures and change, media-use habits, and the like, have been demonstrated to be effective under certain circumstances, and ineffective under other, more or less clearly delineated ones.
- In particular, differential strategies, derived from such notions as cognitive balance theory (e.g., Festinger, 1957) or psychological inoculation (e.g., McGuire, 1964; Pfau and Kenski, 1990), have been identified and evaluated under differing conditions defined by characteristics of extant news portrayals of the image-object in question, and relevant case studies illustrating several such conditions have been developed.
- Increasing numbers of governments are coming to appreciate the potential utility of taking a more strategic view of their external communications. This assertion is supported by both aggregate statistics on such activity and by a small number of case studies of decision making in such countries as Nigeria, the Philippines, Pakistan, and South Korea.
- Specifically, many governments around the world (roughly 160 according to the most recent Department of Justice foreign agent registration records), in addition to their own trained staffs of public diplomatists, engage the services of U.S. lobbyists, public relations consultants, and others to assist them in communicating with the U.S. media and public. Some, but not all, of these efforts could

be characterized as having "strategic communication" components.

• Typically, governments with special needs or problems, or with generally negative images, in the United States are the most likely to engage in U.S.-directed strategic communication, but strategies are available for, and employed by, those with positive images as well.

• For a variety of reasons, ranging from the "obtrusiveness" of issues to the economics of newsroom decision making, strategic communication campaigns within the United States can be more effective when directed at issues or actors in foreign affairs than when employed in domestic politics.

• One condition under which the effectiveness of strategic public diplomacy is minimized or eliminated is where the communication strategy itself becomes widely known. In the United States, all such efforts become matters of public record. However, in part because journalists tend to underestimate their effectiveness, these activities are seldom widely publicized.

In the present study, I will explore the structure of foreign-interest representation in the United States, and the nature of the decision making of both U.S. and foreign governmental actors, and of U.S. political consultants who work in behalf of foreign interests, focusing on both the strategic and the tactical aspects of public diplomacy. In so doing, I hope to suggest not only the nature and extent of this type of activity as practiced on a global scale, but also its centrality to our development of a comprehensive understanding of the making of U.S. foreign policy. More than that, I hope to identify particular approaches or lines of inquiry that will be of special assistance in achieving this objective.

In formulating this analysis, I will draw upon a communication-based analytical framework that examines the internal decision making of, and the interactions among, the media, the public, and the makers of U.S. foreign policy, all with an eye toward identifying the opportunities each creates for influencing the process by some interested outside party. The framework itself will be presented in Chapter 8, but the central idea—that foreign policymaking is an exercise in domestic politics and occurs within a system that is open to purposeful and informed manipulation using basic social scientific knowledge—will illuminate the presentation from the outset.

Before proceeding, let me note two boundaries that operate to limit the scope of the study reported here.

First, as may already be clear but should be stated explicitly, the emphasis in this book is on strategic communication efforts directed toward the United States by other countries. Though we shall touch, from time to time, on outwardly directed efforts of undertaken by interests in the United States, those activities lie generally beyond the scope of this volume. That is the case primarily because a study of U.S. strategic public diplomacy is worthy of both a dedicated research project and a book in its own right. My efforts to date have been focused almost exclusively on incoming information rather than on this outflow. I must add, however, that the inquiries I have made over the years, with professionals at the United States Information Agency and at other points in the federal establishment where one might expect such activities to center as well as with outside observers, have led me to the preliminary conclusion that, when it comes to strategic public diplomacy, the United States gives far less than it gets. Perhaps because it feels less dependent on the largesse of its partners in the international system and is therefore less inclined to attempt this form of political management across national borders, or perhaps because it has not learned to appreciate the power of strategic communication as much as some others have, the United States does not appear to engage in these activities either regularly or systematically. There are undoubtedly significant exceptions to this characterization—perhaps most notably through some programs of the National Endowment for Democracy[5]—and the generalization I offer is not intended to indicate that the United States does not engage in *any* public diplomacy. As I have already indicated, it is quite active in this arena. The argument applies only to the sophistication of those efforts that are implemented.

Second, though, as we shall see in the next chapter, a considerable proportion of foreign agent activity in the United States is undertaken in behalf of foreign-owned corporations and other essentially commercial enterprises, the principal emphasis here will be on government-initiated efforts. It is assuredly the case—as Choate and others argue—that corporate interests verge into the foreign policy arena and that corporations have political agendas in pursuit of which they solicit the assistance of American consultants. But such corporations also have commercial objectives in the United States—selling their products and enhancing their profits—and, indeed, these generally predominate. Governments, on the other hand, even when acting in support of their domestic industries, are generally much more focused on policy objectives. A bottom line concern with the process of making foreign policy, then, dictates my emphasis on official entities.

The book has been organized in three parts. The first, of which you have now completed approximately half, sets the stage by delineating the issues to be explored and examining the system by which foreign agents deliver their services. The second presents a series of case studies that have been designed to suggest both the formal context in which strategic public diplomacy occurs and some of the techniques by which it is pursued. The third part presents an analytical model to be used in understanding and evaluating strategic communication efforts, as well as an assessment of the political and analytical questions associated with both its practice and its study.

Chapter 2 presents a portrait of the industry that has developed within the United States for the purpose of influencing American media, public, and elite opinion to the advantage of foreign governmental or corporate clients. The chapter includes an analysis of data from Justice Department records characterizing the level and type of activity undertaken by U.S. firms registered as agents of foreign interests.

Chapters 3 through 6 comprise a series of case studies, based principally on elite interviews with lobbyists, political consultants, journalists, and officials of foreign governments, that focus on specific objectives and strategies employed in image- or news-management campaigns targeted at the United States and, in some instances, at other publics or governments as well. Chapter 3 examines the systematic efforts to assess and manipulate American public opinion—by Kuwaiti, Iraqi, and U.S. interests alike—to maximize support for a military response to Iraq's 1990 invasion of Kuwait. Because these efforts represent one of the most comprehensive of such campaigns to date, displaying many of the defining characteristics of strategic communication, they provide an especially effective first immersion in the objectives and techniques of the new propagandists. Then, in Chapter 4, we will backtrack just a bit by providing an overview of the formal side of one aspect of public diplomacy, visits by a head of state or government. Here we will examine a fairly routine visit to Washington by then-South Korean President Roh Tae Woo. Chapter 5 details a rather more strategic approach to the same type of event, the "political campaign" waged in behalf of then-Pakistani Prime Minister Benazir Bhutto during a 1989 visit to Washington, the objective of which was to obtain military, economic, and psychological support from the U.S. government. The chapter focuses principally on the technique of "framing," on the shaping of public impressions through the careful and deliberate selection of words or images employed in association with a given person or event. Chapter 6 builds on this notion of framing by suggesting that global-scale events are also employed by governments in the expectation of gaining economic or political advantage. Through an examination of the hosting by South Korea of the 1988 Summer Olympics, the chapter considers the strategic role of what I have termed "mega-events," those that are assured of reaching a massive worldwide audience, in achieving national foreign policy objectives, and the risks attendant thereto.

In Chapter 7, I will argue that policymaking in the area of foreign affairs offers a target of special opportunity to those who would influence the policy agenda. The chapter sets forth a system for evaluating the impact that image-management efforts have on U.S. media portrayals of the client country, and demonstrates both the ability of external actors to influence the U.S. foreign affairs agenda and the limits on that influence. Chapter 8 presents a more complete elaboration of this conceptual framework, which I have termed "agenda dynamics," the general purpose of which is to integrate and broaden the applicability of the ideas first posed more than twenty years ago in McCombs and Shaw's theory of agenda setting and Elder and Cobb's notion of agenda building. Agenda dynamics emphasizes the complexity of interaction among the agendas of the media, the public, and the makers of public policy. The chapter will illuminate, in general terms, the institutional structures and decision-making processes that power the policy process, and that, by extension, represent prospective points of vulnerability to external influence or manipulation.

Chapter 9 begins with a recognition that, to the extent that Americans—media, public, and policymakers alike—are, or perceive themselves to be, victims of strategic public diplomacy, theirs is a victimization grounded in self-flagellation. For, although the interests served by these practices are, more often than not, extraterritorial to the United States, the impetus to act, the delineation of strategy, the expertise to act effectively, and the implementation of action plans—all of these are homegrown. The social and political technology of strategic public diplomacy is made in America. Indeed, it is one of our most successful exports on the world market. Working from this base, I will project future trends in the practice of strategic public diplomacy and will consider their implications for the future of U.S. foreign policymaking.

2

The New "Diplomats": A Growth Industry

> The United States is par excellence a country where public opinion
> plays an important role, inspiring, orienting, controlling the policy
> of the nation. Nothing can be achieved or endure without it, and its
> veto is final. It is characterized by the fact that it is both more
> spontaneous than anywhere else in the world and also more easily
> directed by efficient propaganda technique than in any other
> country.
>
> ANDRE SIEGFRIED, *America at Mid-Century* (1955)

We begin our examination of U.S.-directed strategic public diplomacy
by focusing on those individuals and consulting firms who deliver public
relations, lobbying, and other, similar, services to an international clientele. In effect, as I shall argue momentarily, these service providers
constitute a sizable and rapidly growing industry, one built on expertise
in such fields as social science research, mass communication, marketing, and interpersonal persuasion and fueled by significant sums of
money from a growing client base.

Our review is facilitated by the fact that persons or organizations
engaged in these activities within the United States are required, under the Foreign Agent Registration Act of 1938 (FARA), to register
annually with the Department of Justice as foreign agents, to provide
summaries of the activities in which they engage, and to report all
income they derive from such activities. Despite the fact that these
registrations are matters of public record and are summarized annually
in a report to Congress by the Attorney General, this represents the
first comprehensive survey of the extent of such activity or of its structure.[1]

Trends in Representation

The present analysis focuses on the period from 1967 through 1987. The first of these dates was selected because FARA was amended in July 1966 to exempt attorneys and persons acting in the interests of a foreign principal but on their own volition from the required registration, and to narrow the definition of political activity. Much as would the Glickman amendments proposed in 1991 (see note 1), those of 1966 moved the law from its emphasis on affording protection against subversive activity more toward one of protecting (1) the public's right to know of the registrants' activities and (2) the integrity of the governmental decision-making process. The second date selected was the most recent for which summary data were available. Although 1987 data provide the basis for much of the analysis that follows, they have been excluded from all reports of serial data because of a significant apparent anomaly in the reporting of individual foreign agent registrations, which may be associated with the introduction in that year of computerized recordkeeping.

Table 2.1 reports data on trends in the representation of foreign interests for the period 1967 through 1986. These data are based in part on summaries compiled by the Justice Department and incorporated in the annual FARA reports and in part on an aggregation of raw data drawn from those reports. Included in the table are the number of firms maintaining active registrations each year, the number active registrants, and the number of agreements with new foreign principals. We can see that there has been clear and steady growth in the foreign interest representation industry over this period. The number of firms engaged in this trade grew in two decades from 468 to 824. We have information on the number of individuals in their employ who worked on related contracts for only half of the period, but here, too, expansion of the industry is evident. Perhaps most interesting is the surge in agreements with new foreign clients during the last three years of the series. Though not shown in the table, this number reached 453 in 1987.

Unfortunately, early reports in this series did not include financial data. Then, when this information was first introduced, it was reported only on a country-by-country basis. Only since 1977 have the reports included contract-specific financial data. As a result, it is probably more useful to compare the endpoints of the time period for which we have this information—1977 and 1987—than to scout for long-term trends. This comparison shows that, in 1977, total billings for all services pro-

Table 2.1. Representation of Foreign Interests: Levels of Activity, 1967–86

Year	Number of Firms	Number of Registrants	Number of New Principles
1967	468	2,462	–
1968	446	2,654	–
1969	450	2,478	–
1970	452	–	–
1971	462	–	158
1972	–	–	–
1973	496	–	189
1974	–	–	–
1975	555	–	60
1976	582	–	74
1977	631	5,372	118
1978	663	5,709	137
1979	661	6,026	144
1980	664	6,175	131
1981	701	6,736	125
1982	725	7,230	141
1983	731	7,270	135
1984	751	7,430	171
1985	767	7,649	249
1986	824	8,354	281

vided by all registrants amounted to $353,457,000. By 1987, the comparable figure was $425,210,000, an increase of some 20 percent, all of which occurred after 1980.

It is the sheer size of this pie, but especially in combination with its evident stability as a source of revenue, that has attracted the attention of political consulting and related firms, which see it as an alternative to the more cyclical and less dependable business of conducting domestic political campaigns. Among the most recent to eschew the campaign trail, in part to devote more effort to foreign agentry, are Black, Manafort, Stone & Kelly, which altered its product line when it was acquired by the public relations firm of Burson-Marsteller, and the Sawyer-Miller Group, which did the same when it reorganized twice, first to bring in new partners, including former Reagan aide Ed Rollins, a counterbalance to the firm's traditional Democratic leanings, then again when it was merged into another strategic communication firm, Robinson,

Lake, Lerer & Montgomery, which was already active in serving an international clientele.[2]

Though there is a great deal of money to be made in serving foreign governments, most of the consultants who do so have a firm first rule: Get the money up front. The trade is replete with stories of firms that were stiffed by their clients, or even who were caught in changes of government following which the new leaders were unwilling to pay for the activities of their predecessors, some of which may actually have been intended to prevent the new group's coming to power in the first place. My favorite such story is told by a consultant who was working for one of the major public relations firms on the account of an East Asian government. It was her first—and only—international client.

True to the conventional wisdom, the public relations firm had required the client to pay in advance for its services. This was accomplished by estimating, on a weekly basis, the expenses for the coming week, then faxing an invoice and receiving payment over the weekend, so that, by Monday morning, everything was in order. The work would then go forward. Billings were running on the order of $100,000 per week, including expenses.

The account was essentially a commercial one, and the objective was to pave the way for the visit to the United States of a high-ranking trade mission including representatives of all the client country's principal industries. The group would spend several weeks touring American cities and meeting with counterparts and prospective customers. Once the trade mission had arrived and begun its tour, there came a period of two weeks when logistics made it difficult to bill and receive payment in advance. Yet the public relations firm continued to incur expenses. As time passed, the consultant's supervisor began to express his concern with increasing fervor, until, at last, he called her in to his office on a Friday evening and instructed her to obtain full payment by Monday morning or suffer the consequences.

Finally, the consultant was able to establish contact with the leader of the delegation, who had just returned to Washington. He instructed her to meet him in the lobby of his hotel at 11:00 Sunday morning. Though this was unusual, she complied. When they met, he then suggested that they go to his room. The consultant confesses to having had second thoughts about doing so, but with her boss's admonitions still ringing in her ears—and somewhat secure in the knowledge that she was bigger than her Asian client and could defend herself if necessary—she complied once again.

When they arrived in a suite of great elegance—fine furniture and appointments and a view to match—of the sort generally reserved for visiting royalty, the client asked her to sit and wait while he went into another room. When she heard him open a closet, she says, she became just a bit more nervous. Then he emerged, carrying a large and very expensive Gucci briefcase, which he set on the table before her. He opened the briefcase, which contained approximately $200,000 in *blank* traveller's checks, the equivalent of cash. Here, he said. This is for you.

Somewhat flustered, the consultant decided that the appropriate thing to do was to count the money and provide a receipt. But the client would have none of it, saying that he trusted her completely, and that if there was a shortfall, he would make it up. When she then began removing the checks from the briefcase, unsure of how she would carry the portion that would not fit in her purse, the client stopped her, saying that the briefcase—itself worth several thousand dollars—was a gift to her. She then insisted that they proceed to the hotel cashier, who would be asked to count and document the money. That is what they did, though the cashier's interpretation of the request—especially in a city with an active trade in illegal substances—is unknown.

Finally, the consultant asked hotel security to escort her to a taxi, which she then took directly to her office, where she called her boss and then guarded the money in the firm's safe until the banks opened on Monday. Ironically—because of U.S. reporting requirements for any cash transaction in excess of $10,000—the firm had to fill out forms specifying how and why it received this payment, and it was not until some months later, after the transaction had received federal approval, that it had access to the funds.

Patterns of Representation

Though such anecdotes are at once both amusing and enlightening, they do not capture adequately the full range and nature of the foreign interest representation industry. For that, we must turn to the data summarized in the FARA reports on file with the Department of Justice. Specifically, in the balance of this chapter, we will undertake a detailed examination of FARA registrations for 1987.[3] Our objective is to describe for the first time the structure of contracting and service providing in this industry.

FARA-related activities can be viewed using at least three foci, the client countries, the firms providing services, and the actual services that are provided. Tables 2.2 and 2.3 employ the first of these.

Patterns by Country

Table 2.2 reports on *average* levels of activity for all foreign governments and other non-U.S. entities, aggregated by country, for the year 1987. Included are worldwide averages as well as those for selected regions. Among the indicators reported in the table are:

- the number of agents (firms) reporting a contract during the year with a government of, or a corporation or other entity based in, a particular country;
- the number of such agents reporting that they provided information-related services (e.g., public relations, advertising, preparation of news releases) targeted at the general public;
- the number of such agents reporting that they provided political contacting services (e.g., lobbying, representation before governmental or administrative bodies in the United States, certain forms of information distribution);
- the number of such firms reporting that they provided research or other advisory services (e.g., tracking legislation, image research, polling, legal services);
- the number of such firms reporting that they provided services related to generating or supporting tourism;
- the number of such firms reporting that they provided commercial support services (e.g., industry-to-industry contacts, economic development services, direct marketing);
- the total of billings for each country that were determined to relate to political activity;[4]
- the total of billings for all services provided to each country; and
- the percentage by country of total billings represented by activities judged to be principally political in character.

In each instance, the region showing the highest level of the indicated activity has been highlighted in boldface.

The table shows that the 161 countries or other registering entities[5]

Table 2.2. Regional Variations in Registered Foreign Agent Activity: 1987

Variable	All	Africa	Asia	Middle East	E. Europe	W. Europe	Latin America
				Region			
Number of Countries	161	24	19	18	9	25	23
Number of Active Agents	7.3	3.1	15.5	4.3	5.6	12.2	4.6
Number of Firms: Information Services	2.8	1.5	6.3	2.1	3.6	4.4	1.6
Number of Firms: Contacting Services	2.6	1.1	5.7	1.6	0.2	2.7	1.7
Number of Firms: Research and Advice	2.5	1.0	7.4	1.2	0.2	2.0	2.0
Number of Firms: Tourism Services	1.1	0.1	1.7	0.5	2.0	1.6	0.7
Number of Firms: Commercial Services	1.1	0.3	2.9	0.3	0.1	2.7	0.7
Mean Political Billings ($000)	816	358	2,590	1,327	361	603	356
Mean Total Billings ($000)	2,496	594	4,518	1,658	1,579	3,273	2,514
Political Billings as % of Total Billings (Country Averages)	64	81	62	95	41	42	72

employed an average of 7.3 active agents during 1987. More specifically, the breakout by class of services provided makes clear the proportionately great interest of the clients—governmental and corporate alike—in services relating to information, contacting, and advice giving, those that are generally the most explicitly political in character. The average "country" worldwide spent nearly $2.5 million to obtain the services of U.S.-registered consultants, with more than $800,000, on average, being applied to essentially political tasks.

While these summary measures are interesting, they mask considerable variation across regions of the world. Accordingly, as an element of this analysis, I assigned each country to one region, in most cases corresponding with a continent or contiguous land mass. Levels of activity for the more significant of these regions are also reported in Table 2.2. Interestingly, on seven of the nine listed indicators, the countries of Asia show the highest levels of activity. Those who have read Choate (1990) will not be surprised to learn that the activity in Asia was dominated by Japanese interests, which employed 119 separate active agents in 1987 and spent a total of nearly $37 million on registered activities, including $27 million on political activities. But other Asian countries, notably Indonesia, South Korea, China, and Taiwan, were also among the most substantial of the industry's clients.

Table 2.3 lists the dozen most active contracting countries in rank

Table 2.3. Countries with Greatest Expenditures, by Rank: 1987

Ranked by Total Billings		Ranked by Political Billings	
Country	Amount ($ mil.)	Country	Amount ($ mil.)
Japan	36.9	Japan	26.8
Colombia	34.0	Israel	13.2
Jamaica	31.7	Canada	9.1
Great Britain	19.8	Saudi Arabia	5.8
Israel	18.8	Indonesia	5.6
Canada	16.0	China	5.3
Australia	15.8	S. Korea	3.8
Ireland	14.6	France	3.7
Mexico	14.3	Australia	3.4
Bermuda	12.4	Angola	3.2
Bahamas	11.5	S. Africa	3.0
S. Korea	8.6	Taiwan	2.7

order, first by total expenditures for all services, and second by expenditures for expressly political services, during 1987. In comparing these lists, two points are of particular interest. The first is the limited overlap between the two sets of countries. Only five of the biggest spenders overall are among the dozen biggest political spenders. Among these are not only Japan and Israel, but Canada, South Korea, and Australia. Japan and Israel regularly lead the list in political activity, while Canada at the time was negotiating a free trade agreement with the United States, and South Korea was in the throws of domestic unrest in advance of its role as Olympic host (see Chapter 6). These cases notwithstanding, however, the general finding suggests that many nonpolitical considerations enter into the decision to employ U.S. representatives.

The second point makes clearer just what these alternative considerations may be. Colombian interests, for example, typically spend immense sums for assistance in marketing coffee, while Jamaica, Great Britain, Bermuda, and the Bahamas do the same to promote tourism. And the nonpolitical portion of Japan's expenditures alone, principally devoted to commercial services, would qualify *independently* for the top twelve in total expenditures. Indeed, analysis of the data shows that the largest contracts are not generally associated with expressly political services, but rather, with tourism and a small number of commercial activities. Moreover, many commercial expenditures undertaken in behalf of foreign-owned corporations are excluded from the present analysis altogether because they are not covered under the FARA reporting requirements. This is the case whenever a foreign corporation establishes a United States-based subsidiary or partnership to carry out its marketing, consumer research, public relations, or government relations activities. Such entities are not required to register with the Department of Justice because they are treated, under U.S. law, as American corporations entitled to full corporate citizenship.

The implication of this analysis, that the significance of expenditures for such political activity should not be overstated, is clear. But neither should it be understated, for—in contributing to the general image of a given country that is held by the public, the media, or the political elite and that, as a result, establishes the psychological environment in which policy decisions about that country will be made—the research and promotional activity associated with tourism and commerce is itself not without potentially significant political impact. The import of these image environments will become fully apparent in Chapter 7.

Patterns by Service Provider

We can add to the insights gained through a country-based analysis of foreign representation by taking a look as well at some aspects of the structure of the industry that represents foreign interests. An example is provided in Table 2.4.

Table 2.4 details the degree of concentration of foreign interest representation by the service-providing companies based on reports filed in 1987.[6] In all, 905 companies were reported to have provided services to some 1,514 clients, for an average of 1.67 clients per company. Clients are defined here in country aggregates rather than individually—that is, services are treated as if they were provided to the country in question as a single contracting entity.

What we find when we examine the numbers that lie behind this table is that, while some 80 percent of all companies in this industry have only one client, 41 companies (4.5 percent of the total) hold 27 percent of the contracts, and 107 companies (11.8 percent) hold 42 percent of the contracts. There is, then, both substantial entrepreneurial activity and a noticeable degree of concentration. Among those companies serving clients in more than ten countries in 1987 were: Arnold & Porter (legal services); APCO Associates (public affairs affiliate of Arnold & Porter); Black, Manafort, Stone & Kelly (public affairs); Daniel J. Edelman (public relations); Dow, Lohnes & Albertson (legal services); Hill and Knowlton (public relations); Imported Publications (distribution services); Keating Group (public affairs); Tweed Milbank (legal services); Modern Talking Pictures (distribution services); North American Precis Syndicate (press release service); O'Connor & Hannon (legal services);

Table 2.4. Distribution of Contracts Among Firms: 1987

Number of Companies with . . .	Number of Contracts
720	1
78	2
36	3
30	4
16	5–7
14	8–10
8	11–20
3	21–25

Patton Boggs & Blow (legal services, public affairs); Marilyn Perry; Public Service Audience Planners; Leah Siegel (distribution of news photos); Tromson Monroe Advertising; and White & Case (legal services). It is especially interesting to note that the vast majority of these firms provide explicitly political services. In the context of our analysis of overall industry structure as reported in Table 2.4, this suggests that the concentration of *political* representation may be much greater than that characteristic of the industry overall.

Hill and Knowlton Public Affairs Worldwide

One of the most active purveyors of consulting services to foreign clients in recent years has been Hill and Knowlton Public Affairs Worldwide. In the next chapter, we will examine in considerable detail an example of the company's wares. For the moment, however, let us use Hill and Knowlton to highlight the nature of the consulting companies themselves.

Among the hundreds of firms providing U.S.-directed public affairs services to international clients, Hill and Knowlton Public Affairs Worldwide is perhaps the most prominent and most comprehensive. Founded by John W. Hill in Cleveland, Ohio, in 1927 (Donald Knowlton was brought in as a partner a few years later), Hill and Knowlton today employs some nineteen hundred people in sixty-five offices in twenty-four countries worldwide, and serves more than a thousand clients, including more than half of the *Fortune* 100. It maintains a networking relationship with forty-eight additional U.S. firms and twenty overseas, the net effect of which is to extend its reach nationwide and into some sixty-eight countries. The company's total revenues in 1989 reached $164 million, nearly four times their 1981 level. By any measure, Hill and Knowlton is a major player in international public relations and public affairs.

Even in the 1960s, Hill and Knowlton was established as a leader in the international practice of public relations. Indeed, the firm went so far as to publish a two-volume guide to public relations around the world, with chapters contributed by various of its officers (Hill and Knowlton, 1967, 1968). During the 1970s and into the 1980s, the company continued to develop both its expertise and its services.

In 1986, Hill and Knowlton embarked on a series of acquisitions, which served to solidify its prominence in an industry that is in the midst of a more general period of consolidation. Among those firms which it has acquired in the last decade are:

- Gray and Company Public Communications International (1986), a major international force at the time (its Georgetown headquarters building was dubbed "The Power House");
- Carl Byoir & Associates (1986), at the time the third-ranking public relations firm (and once known for representing German tourism during the Hitler years);
- Timmons and Company (1989), a prominent Washington lobbying and government relations firm; and
- Wexler, Reynolds, Fuller, Harrison and Schule (1990), yet another well-known public affairs firm.

In 1987, Hill and Knowlton itself was acquired by Great Britain's WPP Group PLC, a worldwide holding company (Hill and Knowlton, 1990; Matlack, 1991). In addition to its own holdings, the firm is linked through WPP Group to several New York and Washington "cousins" in the same line of work, including Charls E. Walker Associates (lobbying); Powell Adams and Rinehart (public relations), and Ogilvy & Mather Worldwide (advertising) (Matlack, 1991: 1159). Tables 2.5 and 2.6 summarize the nature and extent of the firm's activities in behalf of a number of international clients.

Table 2.5, reproduced from the company's own promotional materials, summarizes the services Hill and Knowlton provided to some thirty-three foreign governments or interests during 1987. Most significant among these, as measured by the number of clients engaging the service, were communication strategies, international media relations, issue and media monitoring, issues management, and special events, in that order.

Drawn from the Department of Justice's foreign agent registration records for 1987 (Attorney General of the United States, 1988), Table 2.6 summarizes some twenty-one contractual relationships between Hill and Knowlton and various foreign interests, including the contracting agency, the services provided, and, where available, the associated billings. Hill and Knowlton was one of only three firms in 1987 (out of more than 800) to provide services to clients representing more than twenty countries. Unofficial, but more recent, figures show that between November 10, 1990, and May 10, 1991, Hill and Knowlton received

Table 2.5. Hill and Knowlton Services to Foreign Governments and Interests

Country	Communication Strategy	Economic Image Development	Export Promotion	Investment Promotion	Tourism Promotion	International Media Relations	Issues Management	Special Events	Promotional Materials	Issues/Media Monitoring
Alberta/Canada										◆
Angola	◆									
Austria			◆						◆	
Baden-Wurtemmburg/Germany	◆	◆	◆	◆		◆		◆	◆	
Bermuda	◆	◆	◆		◆	◆	◆	◆		
Canada							◆	◆		◆
Cayman Islands								◆		◆
Cote d'Azur/France		◆		◆		◆	◆	◆		
Denmark	◆			◆		◆	◆	◆	◆	
Ecuador	◆	◆								◆
Germany	◆									◆
Guatemala					◆					◆
Haiti	◆	◆	◆	◆		◆	◆	◆	◆	◆
Hong Kong					◆	◆	◆		◆	
Hungary						◆	◆			◆
Iceland	◆	◆			◆	◆	◆	◆		◆

Country	21	13	9	9	8	21	19	19	14	20
Indonesia	◆	◆	◆	◆		◆	◆	◆	◆	◆
Japan	◆		◆			◆	◆	◆	◆	◆
Korea	◆					◆	◆	◆		◆
Kuwait	◆					◆	◆	◆	◆	◆
Malaysia			◆			◆	◆	◆		◆
Mexico	◆	◆	◆		◆	◆	◆	◆	◆	◆
Morocco	◆	◆	◆			◆				
Netherlands	◆	◆	◆	◆			◆			
Philippines		◆		◆	◆	◆	◆	◆		◆
St. Lucia					◆			◆		
Thailand	◆	◆		◆	◆					
Turkey	◆			◆		◆	◆	◆	◆	◆
Vatican City										
Venezuela	◆					◆	◆	◆	◆	◆
Yemen Arab Republic	◆	◆				◆	◆			
Yucatan/Mexico	◆	◆		◆	◆	◆	◆	◆	◆	◆
Yugoslavia	◆					◆	◆	◆	◆	
No. of Clients Using Service	21	13	9	9	8	21	19	19	14	20

Source: Adapted from "Hill and Knowlton: Capability Experience With Foreign Governments and Interests," an unpublished company document dated October 4, 1990. The source does not make clear the time period covered by the reported data.

Table 2.6. Contract Profile: Hill and Knowlton, 1987

Country	Billings ($000)	Contract with . . .	Services Provided
Bermuda	487	Department of Tourism	media relations
Canada	76	Asbestos Institute; Forest Industries Council; Fisheries Council; National Sea Products Ltd.	monitored developments re: marine mammals, fishing, animal rights, environmental activists, seafood inspection; House and Senate contacts; produced radio program
China	–	China Media Services	contacted TV stations to arrange meetings with client
Colombia	–		registered but inactive
Great Britain	44	Royal Ordnance	registered but inactive
France	643	Airbus Industrie; Bureau National Interprofessional de Cognac; Euromissile; Free Trade Defense Association; others	DOS, DOC, USTR contacts re: European aircraft subsidies; monitored trade hearings; arranged interviews; ads and op eds and radio program to oppose import duties; press briefings; marketing advice; general public relations
Germany (West)	–	National Tourist Office	radio program for German-American Day
Hong Kong	148	Tourist Association	arranged press visits, press releases
Iceland	102	Ministry of Foreign Affairs	arranged press visit; monitored developments re: marine mammals, fishing, animal rights; monitored DOC hearings; contacted national security

Country		Clients	Activities
Indonesia	2,186	Batam Industrial Development Authority; National Development Information Office	advisor and others about whaling restrictions and trade retaliation investment seminars, brochures; media relations; news of U.S. economic policy; lobbying regarding U.S. legislation affecting Indonesian exports; produced bimonthly newsletter
Japan	667	Brother Industries; Electronic Industries Association; Hitachi America; Hitachi Ltd.; Makita USA; NEC; Toyo Kogyo	media relations related to plant openings and to legislation; contacted House Appropriations Committee staff and OMB; monitored trade hearings; arranged meetings with Congress and administration on tariff issues; monitored mark-up of trade legislation; direct lobbying
Korea (South)	229	Daewoo; Samsung; Goldstar; Electronics Industry Assoc.; Hyundai	general public relations; contacted House and Senate on auto industry trade developments
Mexico	1,661	Dept. of Economic Development (Yucatan State); FONATUR; Government Tourism Office	planned promotional visit to United States; media relations; promoted new resort; organized journalists' visits to Mexico; monitored publications; wrote releases and features
Malaysia	16	Malaysian Airline System; Palm Oil Registration & Licensing Authority	produced TV series; media tour; wrote position papers on palm oil and lobbied USTR, DOC, DOA, DOS, NIH, House and Senate

Table 2.6. Contract Profile: Hill and Knowlton, 1987 *(continued)*

Country	Billings ($000)	Contract with . . .	Services Provided
Netherlands	97	Central Bureau of Fruit & Vegetable Auctions; Commodity Board of Ornamental Horticulture	monitored legislation and regulatory activity; contacted on fruit and vegetable exports, pesticide tolerances, food labelling and inspection standards, plant quarantine regulations
Peru	–	Minpeco S.A.	press kit for lawsuit relating to 1979–80 silver market scandal
Saudi Arabia	–	Adnan Kashogi	none reported
Spain	24	National Tourist Office	press releases and media contacts
St. Lucia	44	Tourist Board	media contacts, media trips; monitored U.S. media
Switzerland	122	Société Générale de Surveillance, S.A.	information gathering and lobbying re: trade legislation; other government contacts re: inspection regulations
Turkey	1,022	Republic of Turkey	contacts with Congress, DOD, DOS staffs re: foreign aid bill and other legislation; prepared monthly newsletter; wrote two position papers on security assistance for Turkey

Total Reported Billings, 1987: $ 7,568,000

some $14 million in fees and expenses from thirty-one foreign clients (Anonymous, 1991b). It is not accurate to characterize Hill and Knowlton as somehow typical of firms in this industry. Indeed, its list of twenty-one clients ranks third among all firms, and that alone renders it unrepresentative. By the same token, however, Hill and Knowlton offers an array of services that, by their very diversity, suggest much about the nature of the activities that are captured in the data reported in this chapter. For that reason, the table seems worthy of consideration.

Patterns by Activity

Having focused our attention on the representation of foreign interests, first with an eye toward the client countries and then with one toward the consultants providing the services, we must cast our glance in one more direction before our analysis can be regarded as truly comprehensive. What remains is to examine the distribution of representational activities themselves, that is, to look at the number of countries that contract for each of the various classes of available services. Figure 2.1 provides an example of this type of analysis.

Figure 2.1 summarizes the relationship between political billings and total billings for all services. Essentially, the figure asks two questions: Of all the money spent (in 1987) by a given country, what percentage was expended for expressly political services? How did this level of political activity vary across the many contracting countries? To answer the first question, the horizontal axis in the figure reports the proportion, on a country-specific basis, of overall expenditures that was devoted to political activity. To answer the second, the Y-axis reports the number of countries characterized by each corresponding level of political activity. When we put the two together, we find what is termed a "bimodal" distribution—one that has two "peaks"—with the greatest concentrations of countries falling, in this instance, at the extremes of the distribution. Moreover, of the two peaks, substantially the greater one falls between 90 and 100 percent of expenditures.

This figure tells us something very interesting. It tells us that countries tend not to approach *political* activity in the United States in a haphazard manner. Either they make a de facto decision not to engage in such activity to a significant degree, or they decide to concentrate their efforts in the political sphere. It is also clear—from additional analysis of the data underlying the figure—that the cluster at the higher range of

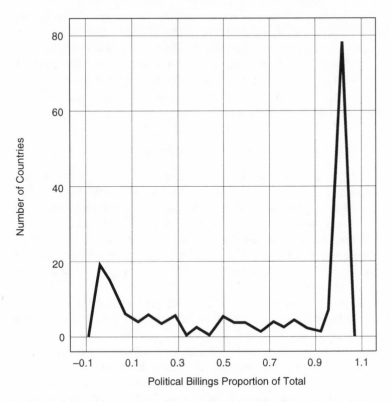

Figure 2.1. Political billings proportion of total: Distribution by contract countries, 1967

activity includes a number of relatively small players who have adopted a selective strategy for employing their limited resources. A few examples among many would include Albania, Bolivia, Cyprus, and (in that year) Kuwait. This finding, together with some of the regional variations noted above, suggests potentially interesting avenues for further inquiry.

Appendix A presents some more specialized results that can further enrich our understanding of the dynamics of foreign-interest representation. Figures A.1 through A.5 employ identical scales to summarize the number of countries engaging in differing levels of contracting for each of five classes of services: Advice/Research, Lobbying, Information,

Commerce, and Tourism. Viewed in relation with one another, these figures clarify the relative importance of each type of service as indicated by *the number of contracts signed.* And they make clear the centrality of services most closely related to political activity.[7]

Other Trends

Two additional patterns in the representation of foreign interests are worthy of note before we conclude, though for the moment neither can be said to constitute a trend. In different ways, each relates to a blurring of the line between what constitutes foreign interests as opposed to domestic ones. Each is best captured through an overview of its most prominent exemplar.

The first of these arose from an incident, uncovered in 1987, in which Toshiba Machine Company of Japan and Norway's Kongsberg Vaapenfabrikk, which were licensed by the Pentagon to produce submarine propellers using a secret sound-damping technology, sold the technology to the Soviet Union, which was then able to reduce what had been a substantial U.S. lead in the ability to locate opposing vessels while they were submerged. This transaction represented a very serious breach of security, and its public revelation produced a furious political response in the United States, especially aimed at Toshiba. There were moves—broadly supported—in Congress to ban all sales by the company in the United States, and in June 1987, the Senate, by a 92–5 vote, added specific sanctions to a trade bill then under consideration.

Under this pressure, the chairman and the president of Toshiba resigned, but no other action was taken by the company . . . with one exception. In concert with the Japanese government, Toshiba mounted a campaign to prevent the trade sanctions from receiving final congressional approval. In all, the company spent an estimated $20 million on this effort, which was characterized by its Capitol Hill targets at the time as the most massive lobbying effort they had ever experienced.

What is particularly interesting in the present context, however, was a second, parallel campaign that was waged by *American* interests. Not only did Toshiba recruit to its cause its own 4,000 American workers and state and local officials in whose jurisdictions the company operated manufacturing or other facilities. Toshiba also mobilized the American electronics industry—companies one might have expected to benefit from its elimination from the marketplace—many of whom, it turned out, were dependent on Toshiba as the sole source for important components in their own products. In the face of this onslaught from domestic economic and political leaders, congressional enmity toward the company withered, and in the end, Toshiba was let off with a mere slap on the wrist (Choate, 1990).

The second example focused less on an event than on an issue: the North American Free Trade Agreement (NAFTA). The objective of NAFTA was to combine the United States, Canada, and Mexico into a continental free trade zone, which, proponents argued, would stimulate long-term economic development in all three countries. The agreement was negotiated by the Bush administration and signed in 1992, and its congressional passage was adopted as a goal of the Clinton administration the following year.

In preparation for the pending vote, the government of Mexico, in cooperation with several of that country's leading industrial groups, undertook a massive public relations and lobbying effort to sell the agreement to the people of the United States. A review of the FARA registrations for the period from 1989 through the spring of 1993 by the Center for Public Integrity (1993), a Washington-based organization that conducts investigative reporting independently of the news media, found that the Mexicans had spent more than $25 million on their effort by mid-1993 and planned to spend an additional $5 to $10 million before the conclusion of the congressional debate on the issue. The center identified no less than thirty contracts with U.S. consulting firms valued at more than $100,000, topped by payments of more than $7 million to Burson-Marsteller, a public relations firm, and its subsidiaries. In all, the Center listed 103 separate contracts between Mexican interests and U.S. consultants or law firms during the three and one-half year period under review, the great majority of which related more or less directly to NAFTA.

Though each of these incidents raises questions in its own right—Toshiba's regarding the appropriate use of lobbyists and consultants to represent foreign interests when the national security of the United States has clearly been violated, and Mexico's regarding the proprieties of scale associated with such activities—they share with one another what may be a more fundamental issue. For each in its own way eliminates the distinction between foreign and domestic interests. Toshiba mobilized its own domestic U.S. constituency to sustain its position;

Mexico lobbied in its own interest, but for an agreement whose acceptance was the established policy of the government of the United States. As the practice of strategic communication continues to develop—and as the national economic and political systems of the world become ever more intertwined—one must wonder how long such distinctions as national interest will remain viable.

Conclusions

From this analysis, we have seen that the representation of foreign interests constitutes a large and growing industry, comprising more than 800 firms with annual billings on the order of half a billion dollars. We have seen, too, that these figures may be systematically understated—that the industry may be considerably larger than even they suggest. We have identified the principal companies providing these services as well as their principal clients, and identified and assessed the relative importance of several types of services that are routinely provided. Finally, we have begun to discern differential patterns of national contracting behavior that appear to be associated with either the region of the world in which a prospective client country is located, or the relative level of activity of individual contracting countries.

In the next chapter, we will begin to explore the nature of this business as it is practiced on a daily basis, the types of decisions that are made and of advice that is rendered, and some of the mechanisms by which image consultants ply their trade in the international arena.

II

Case Studies in Strategic Public Diplomacy

3

Image Management: The Real "Smart Weapon" of the Gulf Conflict

> One dimension of power can be construed as the ability to have one's account become the perceived reality of others.
> H. MOLOTCH and M. LESTER (1974)

> We disseminated information in a void as a basis for Americans to form opinions.
> FRANK MANKIEWICZ, Vice Chairman,
> Hill and Knowlton Public Affairs Worldwide (1991)

To this point, our analysis has centered on two relatively abstract aspects of the representation of foreign interests in the United States—the conceptual framework in which such efforts are best understood and the structure of the industry comprising those who provide them. Before I proceed to set forth a theory of interest representation in the making of U.S. foreign policy and to conduct some preliminary empirical tests of that theory, I think it would be useful to establish just what sorts of objectives governments might have in contracting for consulting services and what sorts of services they might receive in return for their money. That is the objective of the second portion of this book, which comprises the next four chapters.

We will begin by examining a relatively recent, especially comprehensive, and revealing example of image management: that undertaken in behalf of Kuwait—in close coordination with the U.S. government itself—in preparation for the American military response to the Iraqi invasion of August 1990. This campaign more than almost any other displays the full range of needs and services, but also the constraints that operate on those who would manipulate the foreign policy process. We will then turn to three more specialized analyses, one that sets forth the mechanics of a fairly typical head-of-state visit, one that examines the manner in which a consultant can manage public and elite perceptions during such a visit to assist a client in gaining a desired policy advantage, and one that focuses on the image-related objectives of governments that sponsor global-scale events. We begin by considering the role of image management in developing a policy environment supportive of U.S. military intervention in the Persian Gulf.

Memories of the event are probably still strong enough—and the impressions of the event sufficiently potent—that each of us can still call to mind a repertoire of images associated with the Persian Gulf Conflict: Saddam Hussein petting a small boy who was a ''guest'' in Iraq. Former Ambassador April Glaspie under what amounted, nearly, to house arrest in the State Department, lest she comment on her final meeting with the Iraqi leader. George Bush trying to redefine the Gulf crisis as a *golf* crisis. The rockets' red glare over Baghdad, and Peter Arnett hanging out the hotel window to describe it. The ''baby formula'' factory, and infants being removed from their incubators and left on the floor to die. Bombs that were almost cartoon-like in their ability to select targets. Protective gear for chemical warfare. Adolf Hitler.

There were, as well, images that weren't—images that might have colored popular perceptions of the conflict except that their distribution was impeded, or at the very least, not facilitated, by those in a position to shape the flow of news coverage—principally officials of the various governments involved on the side of the so-called ''allies'': Eighty percent collateral damage from less-than-smart bombing. Individual stories of individual hostages and their families. Body bags being unloaded for burial in the United States. An official U.S. estimate of the Iraqi death toll. And there were those for which the image managers might dearly have hoped: The emir rushing home to the embrace of a grateful people.

As the art of managing conflict evolves, so, too, does the art of managing the images of that conflict that are conveyed to the populations of the principals, and increasingly, to a larger world audience.

The motivations for image management during conflict are manifold, and they are not, for the most part, new. They include, among others, the mobilization of support among one's own population and the demobilization of support in the opposition camp, the legitimation of one's own objectives and the delegitimation of the opposition's, the empowerment of one's own forces and the disempowerment of those on the other side, the contrast of the potency of one's own forces with the impotency of those arrayed in opposition, and the very definition of the circumstances and objectives of the conflict on terms most favorable to one's own needs.

What *is* relatively new are the array of technological, institutional, and psychological tools available to the contemporary image manager and, importantly, the growth of expertise in the practice of strategic political communication. The technology of image management is that of modern electronic communication generally: highly mobile field packs, two-way satellite transmission, instantaneous worldwide distribution, and the like. The institutional tools include, in addition to outright censorship, the creation and management of media pools, the selective provision of access to sources and events, the selective granting of media credentials, appeals to the patriotism of journalists and news organizations, the conduct of briefings, grass-roots organizing, and other devices intended to govern who is able to report what to whom, under what circumstances, and, most importantly, at whose discretion. And the psychological tools are those typically found in the workbox of the professional persuader. They are, essentially, those devices by which public opinion can be created, shaped, sustained, manipulated, and directed toward defined objectives. We begin by focusing here on the strategies that determined the specific use of these management tools by a variety of parties with an interest in the Gulf conflict.

In the Gulf conflict, there were several direct national- and international-level participants and at least that number of distinctive targets. These included Iraq, Saudi Arabia and the other Gulf states, what was then still the Soviet Union, traditional U.S. allies in Western Europe, Japan, China, other members of the United Nations Security Council, and, of course, the United States. Though we cannot, in the space available, examine the strategy and impact of all of these participants, we can look closely at four particularly central ones: the Iraqis, the Kuwaitis, the Bush administration, and the U.S. military. What united all four was an interest in defining the terms of the conflict (i.e., the cues that would give it meaning in the public mind), and through them, either broadening or restricting the degrees of freedom available to those who would frame the American response.

The Iraqis

Obviously, the principal strategic communication objective of the Iraqis was to demobilize any support in the United States for diplomatic, economic, or military action in response to the takeover of Kuwait. While it is not possible to know the specifics of Saddam Hussein's intentions, two general points seem clear. First, he did set out to manage the Western (U.S.) media with respect to the crisis. Second, his efforts in this regard were generally counterproductive.

At the time of the Kuwaiti invasion, the Iraqis had a recent history of efforts at media manipulation, but one not notable for its success. One incident tells the story. In the fall of 1988, immediately on the conclusion of the war with Iran, the Iraqi army began an offensive against the Kurds in northern Iraq. The Kurds claimed that their villages were being attacked with chemical weapons, weapons that the Iraqis were known to have used against Iranian forces. In an attempt to disprove these charges, the Ministry of Information arranged for foreign journalists to visit the remote outpost of Zakhu, where they would be able to interview Kurds returning to Iraq from camps in Turkey, to which they had fled. Several dozen reporters were flown by helicopter to Zakhu, only to discover that no Kurds were returning. The government promptly cancelled the "photo opportunity" and prepared to fly the journalists back to Baghdad. On the way back, the helicopters landed for refueling at a military base where reporters observed troop transports, loaded with Iraqi soldiers wearing gas masks, driving toward the Kurdish region. And in the end, the government even confiscated dozens of video-cassettes from the foreign journalists to review them for footage of burned-out villages over which the helicopters had flown (Tyler, 1988). The result was rather less than the intended public relations coup.

Saddam Hussein set out from the beginning of this conflict to manage news portrayals of the event. His principal instruments at first were censorship and the taking of hostages, each designed in its own way to manage a flow of information that was meant to continue. Later, as the conflict deepened and the flow proved largely unmanageable, or when, at the very least, the objectives of news management were not obtained, he evicted most foreign journalists.

The hostage story is perhaps the most revealing of the cynicism, and ultimately the failure of understanding, that guided Iraqi propaganda efforts. Recall that several hundred thousand foreigners became unwilling "guests" of the Iraqi regime. Among them were large populations of laborers, principally from the countries of Southwest Asia, but also numerous skilled technicians and managers from the West, including the United States.

The model here was, rather clearly, that provided by the seizure of American hostages in Teheran during the Iranian revolution. In that instance, the Iranians were able to use their captives to take one additional, de facto, hostage, the president of the United States, who was overwhelmingly concerned with, and was politically overwhelmed by, their fate. More to the present point, it is clear that the Iranian government systematically stage-managed the hostage incident to great advantage. The slogans on the walls of the U.S. embassy compound, and on many of the signs carried by demonstrators, were written in English, not Farsi. Major government ministries had next-day delivery of the *New York Times,* as well as critiques of individual reporters and their work provided by observers in the United States. Direct-dial telephone service with the United States provided the government with immediate reports on television coverage of the scene, complete with network-by-network and journalist-by-journalist assessments (Curtis, 1983). And Iranian "students"—an interesting construct in itself—provided daily advance assistance to American camera crews in identifying the most propitious locations and camera angles for each day's "spontaneous" events.

For his part, Saddam may well have intended to go the Iranians one better. He, for example, did not need to rely on indirect observers of media coverage. He had CNN, and his very own correspondent, Peter Arnett, whose efforts he could monitor with an immediacy denied even the Iranians. And he had not a few dozen hostages, but enough to populate a small country. It must have been a rosy prospect.

As matters developed, we did see similarities in the two cases. Media events were staged to emphasize the presence and vulnerability of Westerners held in Iraq, as they had been in Iran. A willingness to appear brutal was manifested in Iraq—though only with respect to captured pilots rather than detained civilians—as it had been in Iran. And even the signs in Iraq—as at the famous "baby milk factory"—were in English, hardly the language of daily discourse.

But what Saddam failed to understand about the Iranian success was that its smallness of scale, not its greatness, was the key. The Iranian hostages were kept in one central and highly visible place and had names, faces, and families. They were grist for the mill of news media conditioned by more than a decade of pressure to shape programming to maximize audience appeal—to focus on drama and personalization, rather than on ideas, in conveying the content and import of world events (Bennett, 1988). The human scale of the roster of hostages, and the simple imagery of the bevy of yellow ribbons, were central to the potency of the Iranian effort. But by inviting so many guests to remain in his native land, Saddam Hussein turned the story from one of people to one of numbers and lost an opportunity. For a linchpin of almost any media-based strategy of image management is the personalization of the story, providing the media with human-interest content that serves one's purpose. And this Saddam failed to do. His especially awkward efforts to redress the loss—which, among other consequences, gave him the appearance to Western eyes of a pederast when he petted a small boy on television in an effort to appear caring of the welfare of his detainees, a gesture that did not translate well across cultures—served merely to undermine further his control of the storyline. In the end, he was left only with the most intrusive and least sophisticated of all news-management options, the resort to extensive censorship and the exclusion of journalists.

Saddam Hussein may also have had a second vulnerability in comparison with the Iranian hostage taking. For it was a central tenet of the Iranian revolution to expel all Westerners from the country. To Ayatollah Khomeini, their lives and safety were literally of no real value or concern except insofar as they could be used to wring concessions from the United States. Saddam Hussein, however, had no intention of isolating himself from Western support or expertise and knew that in the long term his economy would require outside labor. In this situation, not only would threats against the hostages lack credibility, but they might render unwilling to return to Iraq classes of foreigners on whom the country was in some measure dependent. This, it would seem, accounts as well for Saddam's eventual decision to permit his guests to depart.

If the overall implications of the present analysis are to be believed, Saddam Hussein may also have had yet another disadvantage in that he was not advised in his efforts to shape American perceptions of the conflict by any American consultants. It is my understanding that the Iraqi government did actively shop around Washington for a firm willing to provide assistance in the earliest stages of the conflict, but without success. As we are about to see, the same could not be said of those arrayed on the opposing side.

The Kuwaitis

Of the four parties whose actions are under review here, including both international and domestic players, the Kuwaitis and their agents are perhaps the most revealing of all, because they had no real power to influence events. They had only money, and their objective was to use it to create whatever leverage they could on U.S. policy. In effect, this meant that they needed to mobilize American support for their cause and to channel it into military action, which represented their only hope of regaining their homeland.

To this end, the Kuwaitis enlisted the assistance of Hill and Knowlton Public Affairs Worldwide, a firm whose services and clientele we examined in the previous chapter. This was accomplished through what amounted to a front organization, called Citizens for a Free Kuwait (CFK), which spent some $11.5 million in the United States between August 22, 1990, and March 25, 1991, most, if not all, of it provided by the Kuwaiti government-in-exile. Of this, $10.8 million went to Hill and Knowlton Public Affairs Worldwide (Anonymous, 1991d).

Given the firm's prominence in the field, it is little wonder that, within a few days of Saddam Hussein's march into Kuwait, the Kuwaitis marched into Hill and Knowlton's offices, calling on the company to bring its expertise to bear in behalf of the victims of that assault. Actually, however, this was less a matter of chance than of contrivance. On the evening following the invasion, two Hill and Knowlton officers, Robert Gray and Frank Mankiewicz, dropped by the home of the Kuwaiti ambassador to the United States for a visit. While the conversation that followed was most assuredly not a part of the public record, it seems likely that Messrs. Gray and Mankiewicz mentioned to the ambassador not only their interest in coming to the aid of his country and the full assortment of services their firm was prepared to provide, but also the fact that, within the week, Hill and Knowlton's Washington office would have a new leader, Craig Fuller. That was the same Craig Fuller who happened to have served as chief of staff to the previous vice president of the United States—George Herbert Walker Bush. The opportunity to gain an ear at the White House under these circumstances would have been evident to the ambassador even if it was left unspoken.

It was, in the event, not direct representatives of the exiled government of the emir who called at the firm's Washington Harbour offices shortly thereafter, but rather representatives of the newly formed Citizens for a Free Kuwait. Though virtually all of the fees that Hill and Knowlton collected over the brief life of its contract originated with the emir or his government—the group might have been known as Citizens for El Sabah—the existence of the intermediary organization made it possible for the company to disclaim any responsibility for defending that government and to emphasize instead the commitment of its clients to democracy in Kuwait. The government's support for the group came out only after the fact, when Hill and Knowlton and CFK itself complied with the FARA registration requirements.

Citizens for a Free Kuwait included a variety of Kuwaitis in the United States, among them businessmen, political exiles, students, and some who simply happened to be in the United States on vacation at the time of the invasion. All had awakened on August 2 to find themselves homeless. Among the Kuwaiti leaders of the group, and those with whom Hill and Knowlton eventually dealt, were the former Kuwaiti minister of education, Hassan al Ibrahim; Fawzi al Sultan of the World Bank; and Ali al Tarah, cultural attache at the Kuwaiti embassy in Washington. The group soon formed additional branches in London and elsewhere.

Hill and Knowlton's principal on the account was Lauri Fitz-Pegado, at the time senior vice president and managing director of the International Public Affairs Division, a Latin America specialist who holds degrees from Vassar and Johns-Hopkins School of Advanced International Studies (SAIS).[1] Fitz-Pegado, who joined Hill and Knowlton after five years as a foreign service officer, had represented interests in some twenty countries since joining the firm in 1982. Her base of operations was a river-view office dominated by a political map of the world, a collection of State Department Area Handbooks, and a Rolodex worthy of any Washington powerbroker.

In interviews with the author, Fitz-Pegado and Frank Mankiewicz, vice chairman and managing director for public affairs, described the Hill and Knowlton effort as a twenty-four-hours-a-day, seven-days-a-week undertaking, one that Fitz-Pegado characterized as "the project of a lifetime." Though it is generally the case that public relations firms see international clients as providing them with unique challenges, Fitz-Pegado saw this particular client as more challenging still. "We were," she said, "dealing with people who were traumatized. You had to be a bit of a psychologist to get the job done." She found it an emotionally draining experience.

Part of the problem here, from Hill and Knowlton's perspective, was that the clients did not understand the rationale for much of the company's effort. For example, one theme Hill and Knowlton emphasized early in its effort to build a pro-Kuwait constituency in the United States was the relative freedom of Kuwaiti women. Unlike those in Saudi Arabia, for instance, Kuwaiti women were permitted to drive and, the company's materials noted, even served as university rectors. Fitz-Pegado tells, however, of one Kuwaiti spokesman-to-be who could not grasp the purpose of what he saw as a trivialization of the issues. How can you ask me to spend my time talking about women driving, he wondered aloud, when last week my daughter was raped by the Iraqis? More generally, it was difficult for people who had just escaped from danger and were worried about their families to focus on themes and messages. On more than one occasion during media-training sessions, the clients broke into tears.

Hill and Knowlton reportedly engaged in little direct lobbying, but that is not to say that the firm did not employ its Washington connections to the fullest. According to sources at Amnesty International, which later publicly disassociated itself from a claim to which Amnesty had given currency, it was Hill and Knowlton that gave to the group the story of Iraqi soldiers pulling newborns from their incubators so that these could be removed to Iraq. More significantly, the story also made an appearance on Capitol Hill, where a young woman identified only as Nayirah told a hearing of the Congressional Human Rights Caucus chaired by Representative Tom Lantos that she had witnessed this event firsthand. After John R. MacArthur, publisher of *Harper's Magazine,* revealed in a *New York Times* op ed piece the fact that Nayirah was, in fact, the daughter of the Kuwaiti ambassador to the United States, it was also disclosed that Hill and Knowlton had helped to prepare her testimony, which she had rehearsed before video cameras in the firm's Washington headquarters. This rehearsal took place, as it happens, just down the hall from the offices of the caucus itself—actually the offices of the legally independent but closely related Congressional Human Rights Foundation—which had been for some time the rent-free tenant of Hill and Knowton (Krauss, 1992). It is of interest to note, by the way, that the caucus/foundation also received a contribution of $50,000 during this period from Citizens for a Free Kuwait (MacArthur, 1992: 60–61). Similar, though less publicized, testimony was presented before the United Nations Security Council by a woman identified only as a

Kuwaiti refugee, but who later turned out to be Fatima Fahed, wife of the Kuwaiti minister of planning and a prominent Kuwaiti television personality (MacArthur, 1992: 65; Strong, 1992).

According to Kuwaiti doctors and other prospective witnesses interviewed by Middle East Watch, a human rights group, the incident never occured, a position that was rejected by the U.S. embassy in Kuwait (Cushman, 1992: A11; Priest, 1992a: A17). A subsequent private investigation by Kroll Associates—a U.S. firm paid by the Kuwaiti government—found that Nayirah's testimony was based on a single, brief incident, but that perhaps half a dozen Kuwaiti infants were, in fact, removed from incubators during the occupation (Priest, 1992b: A14). True or not, this story clearly affected George Bush, as evidenced by the frequency with which he cited it, including his turn-of-the-year interview with David Frost, and, judging from the floor debate at the time, also influenced several members of Congress when the time came to vote on authorizing a U.S. military response.

Most of the firm's efforts were focused on media training—their clients, who normally dressed in Western-style business suits, were instructed, for example, to change into Arab dress when appearing on television—drafting speeches and scheduling speaking tours, monitoring and analyzing legislative initiatives, distributing video and other materials, and tracking public opinion. Hill and Knowlton maintained a television crew in Saudi Arabia to produce its own video and also provided a channel—the *only* channel—through which video produced by the Kuwaiti resistance was distributed to outside news services and networks. The firm arranged for events in Kuwait to be highlighted during the Thanksgiving Day National Football League telecast (Anonymous, 1991b).

Of the fees received by Hill and Knowlton, Mankiewicz indicated that approximately $2.6 million were distributed to subcontractors, principally The Wirthlin Group, a polling firm based in Alexandria, Virginia, founded by Richard Wirthlin, a long-time White House insider who had served as Ronald Reagan's pollster, and reportedly owned in whole or in part by Hill and Knowlton itself. Wirthlin conducted daily tracking polls on Kuwait's image and related variables, much on the model of tracking polls conducted for candidates in political campaigns.

According to Dee Allsop, the Wirthlin Group's vice president for communications and marketing research and the company's principal representative on the account, polling began with a nationwide benchmark survey on August 20. This was followed with daily tracking surveys from early September through late October, then with biweekly surveys until mid-December, when polling ceased as it became clear that the objective of the overall campaign—moving the United States to act decisively in Kuwait—was about to be achieved. The tracking polls each contained some thirty items and were administered by telephone to 200 respondents. Principal categories of measurement included the mood of the country, levels of support for the president and for U.S. policy in the Gulf, a series of world-leader and country thermometers, and a bank of specific questions on attitudes toward the Gulf conflict. Wirthlin provided a three- to four-page written report on each survey and sometimes briefed representatives of Citizens for a Free Kuwait directly. (Partial results of these surveys are reported in Wilcox, Ferrara, and Allsop, 1991; and Sigelman, Lebovic, Wilcox, and Allsop, 1993.)

In addition to tracking polls, the Wirthlin Group conducted approximately eight focus groups for Hill and Knowlton and the Kuwaitis, including one group of between thirty and forty subjects who watched a series of videos (e.g., interviews and news coverage from CNN and *Nightline*) while their reactions to both spokespersons and messages were monitored electronically. Wirthlin also piggybacked Kuwait-related questions on its quarterly Congressional Omnibus survey of Capitol Hill staffers in October and followed up with a special survey of top staffers in December. Finally, again in December, the firm conducted the first of what was intended to become a series of studies of school children's attitudes toward Kuwait. The objective here was to attract media interest, but by then there was more Kuwait-related action in other news venues, and in any event, the contract was terminated shortly afterward.

A key question in the present context is the extent to which Hill and Knowlton's efforts in behalf of Kuwait accord with, or differ from, the more general knowledge base developed in persuasion-related social science research. In a sense, the question here is one of just how "strategic" the strategists were. It is not possible to answer that question definitively, but we are able to note several points of convergence.

First, the strategic public diplomacy perspective tells us that strategic communicators will employ systematically the theory and tools of social science to manage client images in much the manner these same techniques are used in domestic political campaigns. Fitz-Pegado disclaimed any such knowledge base for herself other than that of an area specialist, saying that she focused instead on the particular circumstances and perspectives of each client. In addition to Middle East area specialists, however, the team of twenty professionals she assembled to serve the Kuwaitis included economists, media relations specialists, foreign policy experts, foreign aid experts, health policy specialists, and, of course, pollsters. And in addition to the daily tracking surveys, message development was based on a series of focus-group sessions conducted in various locations around the country. Speakers were selected and placed based on the results of these group sessions, with Kuwaiti women and the wives of American hostages sent to some locations, men and "business types" elsewhere. Frank Mankiewicz characterized the media effort as operating at the "wholesale rather than the retail" level, but messages were targeted differentially to, for example, the black press and the labor press. Clearly, this was more than a "seat-of-the-pants" operation.

Second, the strategic perspective tells us that public affairs consultants will focus on themes they believe will resonate among the target audience. Here, the initial theme was that Kuwait was the most open and democratic society in the Persian Gulf region. As we will see in Chapter 5, this was a tried and proven approach to the problem at hand. In addition to the emphasis noted above on women's rights, in this early phase of the campaign Hill and Knowlton pointed to the high percentage of its gross national product that Kuwait had been providing as foreign assistance to Third World countries and focused on the clients' commitment to democratic values and institutions, a theme that has been shown elsewhere to have specific persuasive value.

The tracking surveys showed no trend in the level of support for the Kuwaiti government (recall that the government was not, ostensibly, the client) through the period—it remained steady at just under 60 percent. But in mid-September, the focus groups yielded some important information. They showed that the public reacted, not to the themes of democracy and human rights in Kuwait, but to Saddam Hussein. The focus-group data made clear that the critical factor was response to Saddam as the enemy, while Kuwait was merely a symbol of his atrocities. To Allsop and others working on the contract, who set out initially with some fifty prospective messages from which they sought to cull those that reinforced what people were already feeling, this suggested a two-track strategy. The primary theme was to be designed to reinforce anti-Saddam sentiment. The initial themes portraying Kuwait as pro-

Western, a U.S. ally, and a progressive country, were to be accorded secondary, supporting status. Research then turned to finding the best media for this message combination.

Though the Kuwaitis did not seem especially to like the advice they were receiving, they did accept it, and emphasis on the victimization theme was increased. In this regard, Hill and Knowlton helped their clients to avoid one potential pitfall of such a theme by specifically and repeatedly advising them to eschew talking in public about what the United States government should do in response to the crisis. This advice was generally followed, though the Kuwaiti ambassador to the United States did make some public statements that were more direct.

Third, the literature tells us that image consultants will vary their strategy depending on the extant characteristics of the client's image. With respect to specific cues associated with Kuwait and the Gulf, we have already seen evidence of this phenomenon. In addition, some research suggests that visibility-raising informational campaigns are likely to prove most viable where there is low public ego-identification or involvement with a given image object, but where general public sentiment is favorable. In the present instance, Frank Mankiewicz characterized the initial condition as being low in involvement when he described the Hill and Knowlton effort as disseminating "information in a void as a basis for Americans to form opinions," and the Wirthlin polling data showed a substantial level of popular support for the Kuwaiti government. There is no direct evidence from my interviews that the staff of Hill and Knowlton were operating from an explicit awareness of the social scientific knowledge base in this area when serving the Kuwaiti account. To the contrary, they describe their actions as grounded in their many years of experience. But if not theory-*driven,* it does appear that, at the least, they were behaving in a manner consistent with theory-*grounded* predictions, and a significant increase in December in popular support for U.S. military action may constitute evidence of their effectiveness.

Fourth, the literature on persuasion, which we will examine more closely later in this volume, suggests that attitudes can best be created or influenced where a new and discrepant message displays thematic consistency. In the present instance, we know that several interests were represented in the communication environment, and that diverse messages were being distributed. Any one of them might have been rendered more effective if reinforced by another, apparently independent source.

With that in mind, it is worth noting that, one week before Iraq's invasion of Kuwait, Hill and Knowlton had merged with the consulting firm of Wexler, Reynolds, Fuller, Harrison and Schule. It was this merger that placed Craig Fuller at the Hill and Knowlton helm. Fuller's ties to the White House were maintained long after he left the government upon Bush's selection of John Sununu to head his presidential staff, to the extent that he was tapped to organize the 1992 Republican National Convention that renominated his former boss. More to the point, throughout the period in question Fuller frequently visited the White House to discuss political strategy, as, for example, when he attended a November 8, 1990, meeting with President Bush, the objective of which was to help the administration sharpen its message (Mac-Arthur, 1992: 98–99). This provided a unique opportunity for a coordinated communication effort, one which Fuller later told a *60 Minutes* audience he did try to facilitate. As he put it on another occasion, "Getting [the Kuwaitis'] message across was completely in line with the goals of the Bush administration. By helping the Kuwaiti citizens, it was clear we would be helping the Bush administration" (Mufson, 1992).

The Bush Administration

Though the emphasis in this book is on externally driven efforts to manage U.S. foreign policy, the Persian Gulf Conflict was very clearly a case in which there was a confluence of interest between the key external players—the Kuwaitis—and the key internal players—the administration and the American military establishment—and where that common interest produced a remarkably well integrated communication effort. Accordingly, let us take just a few moments to examine the motives and activities of those playing from the inside.

The Bush administration came to the Gulf crisis with a set of lessons learned, experiences, and concerns, all of which helped to shape both its policy and its strategy for mobilizing public support behind that policy. From Vietnam, the administration knew that it would not be possible to prosecute a war in the Gulf without the acquiescence, if not the support, of the American people. From Grenada—the invasion of which, you will recall, came less than a week after the massacre of American marines in Lebanon—it was clear that the government could deflect concerns and opposition with a quick, decisive, and highly publicized victory (see Deaver, 1987: 147 passim). And from the British experience in the Falklands in 1982 (Cohen, 1988) and its own incursion into Panama, which was aggressively shielded from the prying eyes of journalists until virtually all of the action had been concluded and where it was only much after the fact that we began to learn of the hundreds of civilian victims buried in mass graves, the administration learned that it could maximize its freedom of action in such matters to the extent that it could hide that action from press and public view (Sharkey, 1991).

More than that, George Bush came to office as the clear beneficiary of the use of strategic communication in domestic politics. His presidency was the product of a partisan communication juggernaut that had rolled over one Democrat after another, both in electoral competition and in contests over policy and legislation. This is not the appropriate forum for a full discussion of the Reagan-Bush communication strategy, but it is important to consider some aspects of that larger strategy because so many elements of the domestic effort found their way into the strategic management of images in the Gulf conflict.

The Reagan-Bush media advisors had, for example, considerable experience in limiting access to events by national journalists. Ronald Reagan met them principally in the bladewash of his helicopter. Candidate Dan Quayle confronted them in a press conference held, not in a quiet meeting room, but at a giant rally in his hometown. Stormin' Norman Schwartzkoff met them in a tent where the only video available was that he showed on his own VCR. Lesson learned.

But rather than merely restricting journalists' access—a practice that might lend credibility to charges of their unresponsiveness—the Reagan-Bush media advisors had developed an alternative strategy, one that, like some of them, traced its origins to the Nixon administration. Having observed that local reporters were both less skilled and more easily overawed by access to the president and other key policy actors, that local media would give especially prominent play to national stories gathered by their own staffers, that local media increasingly have the technological capacity to cover national and world stories, and that public cynicism regarding national journalists generally did not extend to local media personalities, Republican operatives have developed techniques for granting access to local journalists at the expense of their national-level colleagues (Smith, 1988: 402–12). The former are more easily managed, and objections from the latter can readily be portrayed as products of professional jealousy. This strategy was employed in the

Gulf through the military's Hometown News Program, a large-scale effort to bring local journalists into the Kuwaiti Theater of Operations (KTO) for the purpose, not merely of coopting grateful journalists who received free transportation to the area (DeParle, 1991: A20), but, more importantly, of creating a clutter of uninformed and repetitive questions that would give the military forces both the excuse to limit access to the front and an opportunity to appear patient and open, at the same time that it minimized the likelihood that control over the story might be lost. Approximately 1,500 journalists passed through the KTO during the conflict. As one analyst summed it up, the administration set up a competition, "newspaper against newspaper, network against network, and television against print," not to get the best stories, but to get such items as visas, privileges, interviews, transportation, and access to the troops (MacArthur, 1992).

Most interesting of all in this context, however, was the handling of the "blood for oil" issue. This was a major point of prospective danger for the president in this particular conflict, and one to which he and his advisors were especially sensitive. In 1986, when Bush was preparing his candidacy for the presidency, his advisor Robert Teeter, through Market Opinion Research, conducted a review of Bush's image and came to the conclusion that his negatives were potentially quite high, especially since he was linked in the public mind with two negative cues: Arabs and oil. The decision was made and implemented to remove Bush from the public eye until the latest possible moment in order to give the public the opportunity to forget about this linkage. Bush dropped from sight for many months, a factor that contributed to his wimp image and even to the characterization of him in the Doonesbury cartoon strip as the invisible man. But if wimpdom was a cost of the strategy, it was not without evident benefits. For when Bush reemerged for the primaries, the linkage to Arabs and oil had all but disappeared. Evidence of this is provided by the news coverage of the Exxon Valdez disaster in Alaska, where slow federal action and a reluctance to penalize Exxon were actual policy outcomes, but where little mention appears of the president's ties to Texas oil interests (Manheim, 1991a).

Clearly, blood versus oil—especially in Kuwait—was a definition of events that Bush could not tolerate, especially if, as Wayne (1993: 47 fn.5) notes, his was the first American company to have drilled wells in Kuwait. To his good fortune, though the theme surfaced from time to time, it generally did so without reference to his own ties to the oil industry. When one particularly threatening front-page story appeared in the *New York Times* referring to ''this oily war,'' Bush responded immediately by staging a rally in the parking lot of the Pentagon at which he delineated the many objectives of American policy in the Gulf, none of which, not surprisingly, had to do with oil (Gitlin, 1991).

One final component of the administration's strategy of information control in the Gulf conflict is noteworthy less for its substance than for its longevity. Throughout the period of the war, and through its aftermath, U.S. spokespersons declined all invitations to issue casualty counts for Iraqi military or civilian personnel. The reasons can only be a matter of speculation. It may be, for instance, that the Bush administration could tolerate the ambiguity of being associated with an unknown number of deaths but not the specificity of association with an established count, was unwilling to admit to significant civilian casualties, or merely saw death as more tolerable to the American people when left as an abstract concept. It is clear, however, that it was established administration policy to avoid casualty counts. So longlasting was this aversion, and so all-encompassing, that, when Beth Osborne Daponte, a demographer with the U.S. Census Bureau charged with updating the Bureau's population estimate for Iraq, following established Bureau procedures, released to a reporter upon request her estimate of war-related deaths— 86,194 men, 39,612 women, and 32,195 children—she was removed from the project, her files disappeared from her desk, and she was fired for having demonstrated ''untrustworthiness or unreliability''[2] (Gellman, 1992).

The Pentagon

Finally, we turn to a set of players whose goals clearly had much in common with those of the administration, but who also had some independent objectives of their own—the U.S. military establishment.

Much of the Pentagon's role in news management was explicit and visible. The faces of press spokesmen Pete Williams and Generals Thomas Kelly and Norman Schwartzkopf became as familiar to audiences around the world as the crosshairs on the monitors of the laser-guided smart bombs that locked onto the doors and windows of so many Iraqi targets. But behind the public relations, there lay as well a clear element of strategic communication. One aspect of this is evident in the Hometown News Program, discussed above, one of whose objectives was to provide human interest news that would fill the media and, potentially, divert attention from other issues. Even C-SPAN got into the act here, with approximately twelve hours of original programming devoted to the transporting of one reserve military police unit to the Gulf and its daily life in Saudi Arabia. But there was more.

Even before the Gulf conflict developed, a small staff group called the CAIG (pronounced "cage")—an acronym derived from Chief of Staff of the Army Asessments and Initiatives Group—had been formed within the service that would bear the brunt of any ground combat in such circumstances. The group, comprised of hand-picked uniformed personnel whose collective expertise covered the full range of army activity, was designed to provide quick, quiet, nonbureaucratic management of public perceptions of military action. Its purpose was, in part, to protect the army from the political consequences of what it saw as the potential for erroneous or unrealistic reporting. Two members of the CAIG had served with the National Security Council, and about half a dozen held doctorates. Members of the group were in regular contact with journalists throughout the Gulf conflict, contacts that required neither advanced clearance nor subsequent reporting to superiors. The CAIG employed a systematic strategy developed within an issue-management framework, and, in the words of Lieutenant Colonel James Fetig, special assistant for public affairs to the chief of staff of the Army and the group's communication coordinator, "This was not a loose-cannon operation."

At Fetig's initiative, the CAIG adopted a variant of the immunization strategy of persuasion. The notion of "immunizing" a target audience against messages that might undermine the position of a given persuader was first developed by social psychologist William J. McGuire, principally in the 1960s (see, for example, McGuire 1964). The essential idea is that one can induce resistance to persuasion through the use of refutational pretreatments. As characterized by Pfau and Kenski (1990: 75) in a recent book on the use of inoculation strategies in domestic political campaigns, these pretreatments "raise the specter of potentially damaging content to the receiver's attitude while simultaneously providing direct refutation of that content in the presence of a supporting environment, threaten the individual, triggering the motivation to bolster arguments supporting the receiver's attitudes, thereby conferring resistance." Pfau and Kenski go on to argue that the central element in such a strategy, and the one that sets it apart from simple preemptive refutation, is the use of threat as a motivating factor.

The principal communication objectives of the CAIG were (1) to keep "SNAFUs" in perspective, (2) to preserve the army's credibility, (3) to prevent surprises, (4) to create the "right" first impression and to prevent false impressions, and (5) to "keep everybody sober." Specifically, with such precedents in mind as the Chinese entry into the Korean War, the TET Offensive in Vietnam, and the Beirut massacre, the group was charged with anticipating and averting potential media/public/political relations problems.

To that end, the CAIG adopted an approach to its task that was grounded in an inoculation strategy. This was evidenced in at least three distinct areas: logistics, casualties, and chemical warfare.

With respect to logistics, the army knew that the scope of the undertaking, moving vast numbers of personnel and amounts of materiel halfway around the globe, would be laden with seeming delays and inefficiencies, and knew, too, that the media and the public would, if left to their own devices—not to mention the human interest stories encouraged by the Hometown News Program—focus on gripes from the lower echelons. Accordingly, the CAIG set out to downplay the level of expectations with respect to mobility and preparation. Members emphasized the limitations on the use of force, citing the example of the invasion of Panama, where war did not accomplish political change. Similarly, with respect to casualties, the CAIG set out to assure that people would know that, as Fetig put it, "if we fought, we would bleed." No estimates of casualties were ever put forward, partly because the military planners were so optimistic in this regard that their estimates (ranging as low as 2,000 U.S. deaths) might have set the army up for a resurgence of the Vietnam syndrome of doubt and distrust. In each instance, the element of threat derived from lingering popular uncertainty over the quality of military leadership, personnel, and equipment, an uncertainty to which the military planners were extraordinarily sensitive.

But perhaps the clearest example of the application of an inoculation strategy by the CAIG came in the area of chemical warfare. The army knew Iraq had chemical weapons and had demonstrated a willingness to employ them. And the army knew that, were they employed, they would result in substantial casualties. This was regarded as a real possibility, and one that might undermine the willingness of the American people to sustain any war effort. Rather than ignore or understate the danger, the

CAIG initiated a dialogue with dozens of reporters in which its members brought up and discussed the issue in what they regarded as realistic terms in order to get it on the agenda early and get people accustomed to the threat. For example, when members of the press were deployed to Saudi Arabia, CAIG members selected a small number of prominent journalists and briefed them on what to expect with regard to chemical warfare, what to look for, and on basic information about the chemicals involved. They made clear the army's expectation that it would take casualties if these weapons were used. Even the C-SPAN series included a briefing on protection against chemical agents. In this instance, the threat was explicit and one that every American could understand. It was raised early and often by the army so as to mitigate insofar as possible any negative consequences for the conduct of a war, and for the army's long-term credibility, should use of the weapons be initiated.

We can see, then, that the military's interests were not in conflict with those of its civilian bosses, but were at once more specialized and somewhat focused on securing domestic political support for the Pentagon itself. The implementation of its communication strategy designed to achieve these objectives became very much a part of the image environment in which support for the eventual military intervention was mobilized.

I can also say with some confidence based on an interview with a member of the British military team that was charged with briefing the media in London on that country's planning for and participation in the hostilities that a concerted effort was made to assure continuity not only within governments, but across them. Specifically, the British would schedule their briefings for approximately one hour after the expected conclusion of the Pentagon's daily briefing. They would then watch the American session on CNN and shape their own statements for consistency, before meeting with reporters in London. The paltry yet much-tolerated Iraqi efforts notwithstanding, then, there was considerable reinforcement for all of the messages in the decision-making environment. The official word was by-and-large the only word.

Conclusion

Hill and Knowlton's association with Citizens for a Free Kuwait ended in December 1990, weeks before the U.S.-led counterstrike and liberation. As Hill and Knowlton sees it, the company's effort to educate both its clients and the American people succeeded. The Kuwaitis' perceptions of Americans changed, their political sophistication increased, and over time they were able to do more on their own and, as well, support for eventual U.S. military action was generated. As some Kuwaitis saw it at the time, however, they were paying a great deal of money and getting little in return (Matlack, 1991: 1159). Whichever view one takes, it is clear that the public relations effort continued long after the contract with Hill and Knowlton was terminated, coming more and more under the direct control of the Kuwaiti government as its authority was progressively reasserted. By May 1991, Kuwait had contracts with four U.S. public relations firms, and by June the government had in place an elaborate effort to show Americans the extent of the country's devastation, a plan that included travel to Kuwait by Commerce Secretary Robert Mosbacher, federal and state officials, congressmen, and business executives, variously paid for by the Kuwaiti government, its embassy in Washington, and even, at the Kuwaitis' request, such U.S. companies as Fluor Corporation, with extensive interests in the region (Anonymous, 1991a, 1991c; Auerback, 1991).

The United States (and its allies) did not engage with Saddam Hussein in the Persion Gulf *because* Hill and Knowlton beat a skillful cadence on the drums of war, with accompaniment from both sides of the Potomac River and of the Atlantic Ocean. To make such an argument on political grounds would be to assume naively that public relations effects operate independently of the many historical, political, economic, and geopolitical forces that contribute to the making of foreign policy in the United States. To make such an argument on conceptual grounds would be, no less naively, to assume that public relations effects necessarily play the role of an independent variable at the top of a very long path of media/public/policy interactions. In the present instance, both sets of assumptions are demonstrably false, and in the larger context, neither is central to the essential argument of this book.

But it would be no less naive to conclude, based on the evidence summarized here, that the campaign for Kuwait was without either political or conceptual significance. Rather, its effects were of a different, and perhaps more complex, type. At the political level, the public relations effort, coordinated from the outset with the warriors in the White House, was not part of the process of policy formulation so much as it was a key element of policy *implementation*. It's purpose was not, in other words, to convince the president of the wisdom of a desired policy, but to maximize his freedom of action in dealing with Congress and the public alike in carrying it off. And at the conceptual level, the campaign served as a catalyst—what social scientists refer to as an *intervening* variable—facilitating the bidirectional associations among the media, the public, and the policymakers as they framed policy toward the Gulf conflict.

4

Coming to America: Head-of-State Visits as Public Diplomacy

On the boats and on the planes, they're coming to America.
NEIL DIAMOND, *Coming to America*, 1980

Though the Gulf conflict example we developed in Chapter 3—with its broad coordination within and across governments and its demonstrated effect in helping to mobilize support for war—is certainly among the most interesting of the known efforts at strategic public diplomacy, it is, for that same reason, among the least representative of the day-to-day practice of the image manager's craft. For far more often than not, the issues are more mundane than war and peace, the strategies and tactics more routine, and the effort to implement them both less intense and less dramatic. In the present chapter, we will shift our focus from the extraordinary to the commonplace by examining the dynamics of one of the most frequent occasions of public diplomatic exchange, the visit to the United States of a foreign head of state or government.

Visits by heads of state or government constitute one of the principal classes of events around which public diplomacy is often organized. Elsewhere, we will use head-of-state visits to illustrate some of the lengths to which foreign governments and their consultants will go to shape the U.S. agenda. For the moment, let us take a rather more systematic look at both the symbolic significance and the celestial mechanics of such visits by drawing insight from the October 1989 Washington visit of South Korean President Roh Tae Woo. Our objective is to cast light on the communication aspects of these visits—how they are planned, orchestrated, and conducted with U.S. and domestic media, elite, and public opinion in mind.

Visits to the United States by foreign leaders come in several varieties, including "official" and "state" visits, with full ceremonial accompaniment; "official working" visits, characterized by lesser amounts of ceremony but potentially equivalent working contact with U.S. officials including the president; and "private" visits, where the visitor may be in the United States to shop, to visit with children in college, to seek medical treatment, or for any of a variety of other reasons. In these private visits, the visiting dignitary may pay a courtesy call on the president, but the trip is otherwise outside the purview of the State Department and the White House. Trips by foreign leaders to address the United Nations are treated (by the United States) for diplomatic purposes as private visits. All of these types of visits can provide a locus for media events and other forms of image making.

The Roh visit, which provides our example in the present chapter, was designated an *official working* visit. It came after more than a year of sometimes fitfull moves toward democratization in South Korea and against a backdrop of growing resentment among the Korean people of the U.S. role in the economic, military, and cultural life of its peninsular ally. We will use the Roh visit to explore several aspects of the use of head-of-state visits as instruments of public diplomacy, with particular emphasis on the decision to make a visit, and the planning and actual conduct of the event.

According to Protocol

The Visitors Section of the U.S. State Department's Office of Protocol has a professional staff of fourteen persons, twelve in Washington, and two in New York. These individuals have the responsibility—in consultation with the desk officers who arrange specific appointments, addresses before joint sessions of Congress, and the like—for working out many of the details of proposed visits by foreign leaders and foreign ministers. This is partly a political process and partly an application of bureaucratic routine.

Politically, prospective visits raise two sets of issues: whom to invite and what sort of invitation to issue. The United States is a relatively popular destination on the international leadership circuit, and it is generally not a problem to convince foreign leaders to visit. To the contrary, the problem is more often to limit such visits, which—because of the commitment of time and resources they require under normal diplomatic practice—have the potential to become burdensome, especially for the president. The art of negotiating such visits, then, is often that of saying "no" or "not yet" in the least offensive way possible. Indeed, even when an invitation is to be extended, tact is required in setting the level of the visit, especially where it is not to be one of the more prestigious official or state visits. Since informal departmental guidelines suggest that official visits be limited to two per month, including only one state/official visit and one working visit, the potential exists for half of all visiting foreign leaders to take offense. Though these decisions may seem rather mundane, they become, in effect, a significant element of *American* public diplomacy, communicating to foreign leaders and peoples alike messages about their relative centrality to the American world view.

And the decisions are of some moment. Governments often lobby very hard to obtain the highest status for their leader's visits or to have lesser visits supplemented by special events (typically involving the president). This lobbying has prompted one official to describe the embassies in Washington—and even some State Department desk officers—as displaying "client-itis," a drive to get all they can for their prospective visitor. In effect, they are competing with one another for the political benefits a visit can bring.

We can begin to understand the reasons for this competitiveness by considering the "standard packages" that the State Department—in close consultation with the White House—offers to visiting dignitaries. As the term suggests, the department serves in such instances as, essentially, the nation's tourist office of highest resort, and in some ways its role is best understood by pursuing that analogy.

At the top of the prestige ladder are the state and official visits. *State visits* are accorded only to heads of state (e.g., monarchs, presidents), while *official visits* are accorded to heads of government (e.g., prime ministers). They differ only in minor degree. State and official visits to the United States include a stop at the White House that always begins at 10:00 A.M. with a welcoming ceremony on the south lawn replete with full military honors, the playing of both national anthems, a review of the assembled troops, a presidential welcoming statement and a response by the visiting leader. A translation of the president's remarks is whispered in the ear of a visitor who does not understand English, while his or her remarks in a language other than English are translated publicly. The entire (official) visiting delegation—which always numbers fourteen (regardless of how many additional persons may actually have accompanied the visitor) and includes the visitor's spouse and the country's ambassador to the United States and his/her spouse—participates in the ceremony, which receives full press coverage. The welcoming ceremony is followed at 10:30 with a reception in the White House attended by such persons as the dean of the diplomatic corps, the secretary of state, and the chairman of the joint chiefs of staff. This is followed in turn by a private meeting of some fifteen minutes duration with the president in the Oval Office, an expanded meeting directly afterward in the Cabinet Room just across the hall of the West Wing including the president, the visitor, and seven additional representatives of each side, and, often, a luncheon with the secretary of state at the State Department.

Dignitaries who are guests of the United States for state and official visits may stay for not more than three nights in Washington (at Blair House, the official guest residence) and an additional three nights elsewhere. Blair House can accommodate up to fourteen people (including spouses, security personnel, valets, doctors and others, as well as the official visitor) and may be host to no more than one visitor at a time, so most of the retinue will find accommodations elsewhere (typically at a nearby hotel). Other highlights of such visits include a state dinner at the White House, a departure ceremony on the grounds of the Washington Monument featuring an artillery salute (twenty-one guns for a head of state and nineteen for a head of government), and a helicopter ride from there to Andrews Air Force Base. For heads of state who do not have their own aircraft, the United States may provide a presidential jet to carry a party of up to twenty-one persons from the U.S. city of embarkation (typically New York for those arriving via their national airline) to Washington, and from there to one U.S. destination. All heads of state or government are protected by the U.S. Secret Service for the duration of their stay and are provided with interpreters skilled in simultaneous translation.

An *official working visit* comes with fewer perquisites. The visitor is still an official guest of the United States and is afforded the many courtesies that entails, but on a less grand scale. Those on a working visit may form an official delegation of only twelve persons and are entitled to only two nights in Blair House. They receive no formal arrival ceremony at the White House, but do pass through an honor cordon in the West Lobby. They have a fifteen-minute personal meeting with the president in the Oval Office and a forty-five minute expanded meeting similar to those afforded state visitors, as well as a working luncheon with the president in the old family dining room, all followed by departure statements by the president and the visitor. It is also customary for such visitors to have lunch at the State Department on their last day in town. Those on working visits do not receive a gun salute on departure, but may receive one if they lay a wreath at Arlington Cemetery. (An Arlington visit is one of several "options" the State Department makes available for those who want to add ceremony to their visits.)

In effect, the choice offered to visiting chief executives is between ceremony and substance. The state and official visits offer more of the former, including ample photo/video opportunities, and appear to carry more prestige. Working visits, on the other hand, command more "quality time" with the president.

Those coming to the United States on *private visits* are not considered guests of the government, but may be offered protective security (this is not automatic) or other considerations of an official nature. As noted, they may schedule courtesy visits with the president, but these are generally brief and informal.

If we view these "standard packages" from the perspective of a foreign leader interested in communicating messages either to the U.S. public or to a domestic one, we can see that more than just prestige is at stake in determining the status of a forthcoming visit. Photo opportunities, sound bites, and the other trappings of newsworthiness—and the chances they offer to guide or control the United States or domestic news agenda—vary greatly depending on the class of one's travel, regardless of whether the objective is to highlight a Washington visit or to obscure it. Small wonder, then, that governments lobby the State Department to upgrade or in some other way customize their leader's visit. Indeed, such lobbying can be quite intense. And it is in response to that fact, and to the need to accord the equivalent treatment to all visiting leaders that diplomatic convention requires, that the department has fallen back on the bureaucratic style reflected in its standardization of the process. In effect, the routinization of the process, and the great reluctance of the department to vary significantly from the standard packages, has been adopted precisely to provide a diplomatically defensible rationale for all decisions regarding visits.

The President Is Coming!
The President Is Coming!

From most accounts, at least those of people who work at them, foreign embassies in Washington are seriously understaffed. Whether in the political section or the press office, most of the diplomats and other embassy personnel I have talked with over the years have complained of workloads and expectations far in excess of their departments' capacities. Leaving aside a few major embassies, for example, a professional staff of one to three persons might typically be charged with monitoring all U.S. news coverage of their country, briefing the Washington political officers and the home government on American media and public opinion, establishing and maintaining relationships with U.S. journalists and educating them about the country and its interests, responding in a timely manner to media inquiries, and engaging in various forms of public relations and outreach activity. Add to this the occasional crisis or a rising level of American interest in a given country, and the job can become quite overwhelming. Yet the policy interests of a government—some of them very substantial—can depend heavily on the right or wrong word being said in the right or wrong place by or to the right or wrong person. For those many countries who view their relations with the United States as important to their national interest, the pressure on the diplomatic corps can be intense.

But all of this pressure pales by comparison with the situation that arises when the boss comes to town. Suddenly the workload doubles, for in addition to all of the above-listed responsibilities (or their equivalent in other areas of embassy operations), the same staff—typically without significant additional assistance, though, as we shall see in the case of Ferdinand Marcos's 1982 visit, there have been exceptions—must also manage an event of great significance. They must attend to scheduling, security, social amenities, diplomatic niceties, and a surprising number of basic housekeeping chores that arise only because the president, prime minister, or monarch is on the way. And it is, after all, the CEO who is coming, the great appointer and dismisser, promoter and demoter. Those who do their jobs singularly well can hope for attention, while those who do not can only hope to avoid it.

As noted, heads of state or government travel for a variety of reasons, many of them personal and private. For present purposes, however, we shall focus only on official travel. Viewed from the domestic side, official foreign travel by the national leader becomes a focal point of media and public attention. When domestic issues become especially contentious and the symbols of political exchange emphasize divisions in the society, for example, overseas travel can be used to renew a sense of commonality and to generate feelings of national unity. And when things are going well, such travel can become a symbol of national pride. Travel by a national leader, then, can be seen as a significant event that can, at least potentially, be timed and managed for its maximal political benefit.

Viewed from the foreign policy side, visits to one's negotiating partners can serve a number of purposes. Such travel, or the issuance of an invitation to visit, is a sign of respect—it connotes the importance that one nation attaches to its relationship with another. It can facilitate the conduct of negotiations on such diverse topics as trade, military bases or alliances, cultural exchanges, or human rights. It can break down barriers through the establishment of personal relationships—arguably a primary benefit of the now commonplace summitry between the United States and Russia or among the leaders of the so-called G-7, the major industrial nations. It can communicate to the world (or to the citizens of the participant states) an appearance of concern, unity, friendship, progress in resolving disagreements—even where none exists. It can provide opportunities for credit claiming—for example, for signing treaties that lower-ranking diplomats have negotiated, perhaps over many years. Or it can serve as one of the techniques by which the government of one country appeals to the citizens of another to view it in more positive (or, perhaps, less negative) terms. Even where such visits have specific policy agreements as their primary objective, no government can afford to overlook their secondary effects as instruments of public diplomacy. And it is those effects, and the efforts directed toward them, that provide the focal point of the present analysis.

The View from "Over There"

Roh Tae Woo was elected to the presidency of the Republic of Korea in 1988 in the midst of a political and social upheaval of near-revolutionary proportions. In the wake of the assassination of President Park Chung Hee in 1979, South Korea had entered into a period of political instability that reached a nadir on May 26, 1980, when military forces led by then-General Chun Doo Hwan violently suppressed student and other demonstrators in the city of Kwangju. On June 4, the United States dispatched a naval force to Korea in support of Chun, and on June 5 a new, de facto government was formed. On September 2, 1980, Chun Doo Hwan was inaugurated as president of the Republic of Korea. Casualty reports of the Kwangju incident have varied widely over the years (the original government claim was that some 200 persons had been killed, while others claimed the number was ten times as high), but the one constant product of the battle in the streets of the provincial capital has been a residue of bitter and animated distrust of the government among some Koreans over all the years since.

During the 1980s, the Chun administration developed a reputation for authoritarian rule that was reinforced by a series of actions targeted at leaders of the political opposition. During this same period, however, the economic opportunities available to Koreans expanded rapidly as the country emerged as a major player in world trade. This new affluence led to a rising tide of political expectations that the government was slow to appreciate and culminated, in the spring and summer of 1987, in a series of stylized street clashes between students—the traditional harbingers of political change in Korea—and the government's army of riot police. Roh Tae Woo, President Chun's designated successor, and at the time widely regarded as something of a political lightweight, established the legitimacy of his claim to national leadership literally overnight when he delivered a speech in which he appropriated the agenda of the opposition as his own and assumed the mantle of the political reformer. In subsequent years, he demonstrated a penchant for compromise that was, in a sense, distinctly un-Korean, but that, as a tactical device, allowed him to keep the opposition off balance and to maintain his own authority. The transition to civilian democracy was then concluded when President Roh yielded his office to President Kim Young Sam, long a leader of the opposition forces, in 1993.

President Roh's 1989 visit to Washington is best understood within the larger context of the Koreans' approach to external communication. I had an opportunity to visit Korea three times during 1987 and 1988 and to meet with many of the officials responsible for conducting that country's public diplomacy. Though the circumstances had changed a bit by the time of the presidential visit in 1989, the players and the general perspectives were mostly unchanged. I would characterize them as follows.

In the view of those officials charged with conducting the U.S.-directed public diplomacy of the Republic of Korea, the salient aspects of Korea's diplomatic situation were that the country:

- was a small country with a growing but unavoidably dependent economy and a highly educated population;
- had undergone a period of rapid development that had generated a crisis of rising economic and, more recently, political expectations;
- had a tradition of bilateral diplomacy in which, historically, it prospered by identifying and accommodating the principal expectations of its patron state, which in this instance centered on the nature and pace of democratization; and
- was confronted on its only international boundary by a hostile and aggressive neighbor, whose presence required the maintenance of a disproportionately large military force and the stationing of a substantial garrison by the protecting power, the United States.

From this perspective, the tasks of the external communications program targeted at the United States were to preserve the willingness of the United States to defend South Korea against aggression and maintain favorable terms of trade with its client state, and to channel the pressure for democratic political development in ways that were consistent with the needs and capabilities of the Korean political elite. In short, the objective was to use external communication to complement other means of achieving economic growth and political stability by fostering a facilitative relationship with the government and people of the patron state.

To this end, Korean public diplomacy was generally channeled through either governmental or quasi-governmental agencies and was targeted primarily, and in approximate order of precedence, at the following groups:

- American political elites, including both current and former public officials;
- American intellectual elites;
- American business leaders (a number of agencies whose mission is to communicate with business leaders lay outside the scope of my research during these visits);
- American journalists, and through them
- the American public.

These efforts were organized into three groups: elite relations, public relations, and press relations.

Elite Relations

Much of South Korea's external communication effort employs interpersonal relations. Through a network of government agencies, affiliated research institutes, and private foundations with close government ties, the Koreans play host to large numbers of prominent Americans each year. Leaving aside business elites, these visitors fall into two general categories: current and former political leaders, and scholars and educational leaders.

The operations of two independent organizations that worked in close cooperation with the government illustrate the nature and extent of these contacts. These included the International Cultural Society of Korea (ICSK), which has ties to the Reverend Sun Myung Moon and the Reunification Church, and the Ilhae Foundation (renamed the King Sejong Foundation subsequent to the time this research was conducted).

The ICSK was founded in 1972 for the purpose of establishing cultural relations with countries around the world. To this end, it sponsors international conferences bringing together Korean and foreign scholars, exchange programs in the performing arts, a personnel exchange program bringing visitors and guest lecturers to Korea, and since 1982, fellowship grants for foreign scholars and researchers interested in Korean culture and related topics. In addition, ICSK maintains a publication and reference service, including the publishing of weekly or monthly magazines in English, French, and Japanese. Its objectives are to portray a positive image of Korea in the world and to provide a forum for expressing opinions on Korean affairs.

In 1986, ICSK programs operated on a budget of approximately $3.4 million, up from $2.2 million the year before. Of this sum, approximately 45 percent was expended on cultural exchange programs (compared with 18 percent in 1985), 8 percent on personnel exchanges (21 percent in 1985), and 21 percent on publications (47 percent in 1985). Revenues came from advertising, donations and contributions (which roughly doubled from 1985 to 1986), individual membership dues (1 percent), and other sources.

From its inception, ICSK activities have focused heavily on the United States. For example, of some 898 individual guests invited to

South Korea between 1976 and 1986, 354 (39 percent) were from North America (almost all from the United States). Among the U.S. visitors between 1983 and 1986 were thirty-three academics (principally in political science, sociology, and communication), researchers at the Hudson Institute and the Heritage Foundation, more than a dozen journalists, the chairman of the board of the Ford Foundation, and one U.S. senator. A similar emphasis on the United States is evident in other society programs. Some 68 percent of all books and 30 percent of all magazines distributed by ICSK in 1985 went to North America, and North Americans accounted for the largest share of honorary memberships in the Society (International Cultural Society of Korea, 1986, 1987).

The Ilhae Foundation was more recent in origin and assumed an increasingly important role during the Chun administration in arranging exchanges with academic institutions and with policy planning groups in the United States. "Ilhae" was the nom de plume of former President Chun Doo Hwan, and it was to the foundation that the president planned to retire on completing his term of office. (In the event, this "honorable" retirement was denied him.) The Ilhae Foundation conducted an annual "home and home" exchange program with scholars at the Center for Strategic and International Studies focusing on economics, security, and politics. In addition, Ilhae had long-standing ties with the Heritage Foundation and each summer sponsored a visit to Seoul by ten to twelve scholars from the Brookings Institution to lecture on economic issues. Korean participants in these programs were almost exclusively leaders in business and government. For example, some fifty business executives typically attended the Brookings lectures.

Both the ICSK and the Ilhae Foundation were private organizations, but both worked cooperatively with the Korean government. In addition, the government itself operates a visitors program through a variety of ministries including, in particular, the Ministry of Culture and Information. For example, the Korean Cultural Service in New York has assisted the so-called Korean Studies Group, organized by the Council on Foreign Relations and including journalists and others interested in Korean affairs, in arranging visits. In addition, The Korea Society, based in New York, brings together business leaders, political figures, and scholars for a variety of discussions, social activities, and other events.

The emphasis in all of these exchanges on identifying and establishing personal relationships with U.S. intellectual and political elites reflects both the personalistic style of Korean politics and what one might term the "proactive clientism" of the country's bilateral relationship with its protecting power. The substantial resources and energy devoted to these contacts evidence their centrality in South Korea's public diplomacy strategy.

Public Relations

In addition to fostering personal contacts with U.S. elites, the Koreans devote considerable resources to more diffuse forms of image making and of influencing U.S. policy on matters of concern. The pattern here is similar to that of elite relations activities in that government agencies work cooperatively with the private sector to achieve common goals. The FARA records of the U.S. Department of Justice show, for instance, that in 1987 some forty-six contracts were signed between the government and other Korean interests and various U.S. firms for public relations, lobbying, legal, and other covered services. The reported value of these contracts totaled approximately $8.6 million. By far the greatest portion of this money was spent by groups like the Korean Trade Promotion Corporation for such purposes as locating Korean manufacturers to produce goods for U.S. companies, circulating trade inquiries from Korea in the United States, conducting market research, arranging exchange visits between Korean economic officials and U.S. business people and local government officials, and resolving trade disagreements.

A significant portion of the overall effort, however, was more directly political in character. In one typical year, for example, Arnold and Porter, a Washington law firm specializing in international trade, provided advice to the Korean Foreign Trade Association on U.S. laws, regulations, and policies regarding trade and taxation and on pending legislation, and lobbied on behalf of the association on tariff matters. Baron/Canning Company of New York advised the Korean government on political, economic, and trade issues, while Gray and Company, a major Washington public relations firm that later merged into Hill and Knowlton, produced a bimonthly report advising Korean officials on bilateral trade issues. Hill and Knowlton itself monitored congressional and executive branch activity on trade policy and steel and textile issues for Daewoo International Corporation, a major Korean manufacturer. And Clyde Gardner Hess of Washington prepared press releases, wrote speeches and letters, and assisted in producing a monthly newsletter, all for the Korean embassy, and provided general advice on the conduct of the embassy's public affairs programs.

As mentioned, one of the principal contracting organizations for lobbying and public relations assistance in the United States is the Korean Foreign Trade Association (KFTA), founded in 1946 and known until 1987 as the Korea Traders Association. The name of the association was changed because the original conveyed an image in the United States of brokers rather than one of producing industries. KFTA is a private association of some 10,000 licensed traders and member companies with headquarters in Seoul and branch offices in Washington and New York (as well as in Tokyo, Hong Kong, Düsseldorf, and Brussels). The association's Washington office, staffed by five Koreans and three Americans, provides its principal link with the United States.

Within KFTA, the Trade Cooperation Department, with 18 staff positions (out of a total of more than 500) has the primary responsibility for monitoring and reacting to trade policy developments in the United States. Established in 1984, it collects information on foreign trade matters and policies and organizes responses to perceived foreign protectionism against Korean products. In the United States in 1987, KFTA employed three law and consulting firms (Arnold & Porter, Malmgren Inc., and Manchester Associates Limited) to assist and advise it on these issues, to monitor policy developments and proposed legislative changes, to recommend countermeasures, and to arrange meetings between Korean government and business interests and U.S. journalists, members of Congress, and others. In addition, KFTA works to improve the image of Korean industry in the U.S. press.

The selection of U.S. consultants by KFTA is especially revealing of the relationship between a variety of private-sector organizations and the Korean government. When queried about the procedures by which the firms listed above were chosen, an official of the association noted that they had been "recommended" by several government officials. The same official indicated that KFTA cooperated with the efforts of the Economic Planning Board (a government agency) to generate a unified strategy for projecting Korea's image overseas.

With regard to public relations and lobbying activities in the United States, then, the organization of programs is similar to that for elite relations in that it involves at least some informal coordination between the Korean government and a variety of private-sector organizations.

Press Relations

Though the Republic of Korea is a major trading partner of the United States and a principal ally on the Pacific rim, few American news organizations maintain a significant presence in Seoul. Those that did in 1987 included:

- Associated Press (5 staffers),
- United Press International (2 staffers),
- ABC (2 staffers),
- CBS (2 staffers),
- NBC (2 staffers),
- CNN (1 staffer),
- Voice of America (1 staffer),
- Washington *Post* (1 staffer),
- Washington *Times* (1 staffer), and
- *Asian Wall Street Journal* (2 staffers).

This amounted to some nineteen journalists stationed in the country, only five of whom (as of June 1987) were not Korean nationals. The foreign press corps at that time also included representatives of Reuters, AFP, DPA, Visnews, the *Sunday Times,* and the *Far East Economic Review*. All together, however, fewer than a dozen Westerners were assigned to Seoul bureaus, and fewer still were fluent in the Korean language.

Under most circumstances, foreign journalists have two points of possible contact with the Korean government. These include the press relations staff of the president and the Korean Overseas Information Service (KOIS).

All information about the activities of the president of the Republic of Korea in 1987 was disseminated by a press relations staff housed in an office building at the Blue House, the presidential residence and compound located on a mountainside in Seoul. The chief press secretary and spokesman for the president headed the press operation. He attended meetings involving the president (often, at least during the Chun administration, as the only third party present), prepared official transcripts, issued official statements, and responded to inquiries. A second official, with the title press secretary to the president, had primary responsibility for dealing with the foreign press and for monitoring the country's image overseas. The secretaries were assisted by a small staff.

My interviews and observations suggested that, at least at the time of my visits, the press relations staff tended to take a reactive, as opposed to a proactive, approach to the foreign press. That is, these officials were more likely to wait for news to come out than they were to attempt to stimulate or channel it themselves. As a consequence of this approach and of the general tendency of Western media to focus primarily on "negative" news of foreign affairs, even during periods of relative calm, they were more often engaged in crisis management and damage control than in news management and image control. One effect of this reactive style is that the press secretaries tended to develop antagonistic attitudes toward the foreign news media and to engage in defensive behaviors that were ultimately counterproductive to their interests.

For a variety of reasons, the relationship between foreign correspondents and the Blue House during the period of my observations was characterized by a high degree of mutual distrust, which made it harder for reporters to do their jobs, reduced the ability of the president's staff to influence the spin of the news, and on balance, reduced the quality of information about Korean events that was published in the United States. One official captured these feelings very well when he described U.S. journalists as engaging in a "structural conspiracy" against the Korean government, a sentiment that was no doubt heightened by the pressure on the government at the time of the interview, but that traced to an earlier time.

KOIS, the second government agency with responsibility for dealing with foreign journalists, experienced a similarly stormy relationship with the press. KOIS is an agency of the Ministry of Culture and Information and is headquartered in Seoul. It has a staff of approximately a hundred in the capital and forty representatives stationed in embassies around the world as press attachés. Next to the Ministry of Foreign Affairs, KOIS fields the largest contingent of Korean diplomatic personnel abroad. Its objective, in the words of the director general for the foreign press, is "projecting the true and better image of Korea overseas."

KOIS is organized into two bureaus, one of which dealt with publications and the other with the foreign press. Some information regarding its organization and activities is classified, but the scale of its operations is indicated by the fact that in 1986 it conducted 21 press briefings attended in the aggregate by 574 correspondents, conducted quarterly press tours for a total of 135 correspondents (e.g., to the Demilitarized

Zone bordering North Korea), and distributed 139 releases to the press (with a distribution list of more than 5,000 recipients).

KOIS serves as the central press office for all ministries and agencies of the Korean government below the presidential level and occasionally for statements from the president as well. All releases are handled through KOIS, and all press inquiries are referred there. The agency provides centralized processing for all news photos taken in Korea and maintains satellite uplink facilities. KOIS helps journalists arrange visas, schedules meetings for them with officials of the government and the various political parties (though most journalists prefer to arrange meetings with opposition party leaders independently), and organizes press conferences with officials of various ministries or the police when events warrant. From time to time, KOIS has also organized workshops for resident and visiting correspondents. These sessions, usually scheduled at resort hotels, include panels with presidential secretaries, ministry representatives, and scholars. Topics included a range of issues in political and economic affairs. KOIS also provides guides and translators for visiting journalists.

Western correspondents are wholly dependent on some of these KOIS services and take advantage of others, all the while maintaining an arm's length relationship. Those stationed in Seoul seem to know KOIS officials and others in the Ministry of Culture and Information well, but at least at the time of my interviews and in some cases more generally, expressed considerable distrust of their motives. These journalists were reluctant to speak openly in the presence of KOIS personnel, and all had stories to tell of their conflicts with agency policies.

The role of the foreign press in pressuring the government for political change in 1987, and the resentment of that role on the part of government officials, undoubtedly accounted for a considerable degree of the apparent animosity between these parties at the time of my visit, but the mutual distrust between the press corps, on the one hand, and the Blue House and KOIS (and other government officials) on the other, traces in no small measure as well to fundamental differences in extant perceptions of the ''proper'' role of the press in reporting Korean affairs. For their part, the journalists perceived that persons in the government were out to protect themselves from outside scrutiny. Applying the skepticism and adversarial approach that typify Western journalism, American reporters saw their role as using the news as a force for enhancing openness, responsiveness, and fairness in a political system, whether that of the United States or of South Korea. And for its part, the Korean government believed that journalists should be willing to report good news as well as bad (a common theme in the debate over so-called "development journalism"; see, e.g., Salwen and Garrison, 1988) and should show greater respect for the position of certain public officials. It operated in a defensive and highly bureaucratized manner that tended to reinforce journalists' initial distrust.

To be sure, some or much of this structure and mind-set may have changed as part of the larger political change that has occured in the Republic of Korea in the years since my visits. They did, however, set the context within which planning took place for President Roh Tae Woo's visit to the United States in October 1989.

The View from "Embassy Row"

As I have already indicated, embassy personnel who are charged with coordinating a head-of-state visit view the event as both a challenge and an opportunity.

President Roh's 1989 visit to Washington came at a time when the domestic political scene had stabilized somewhat, but when little real progress had been made toward resolving the one remaining issue on the agenda of national reconciliation—reunification with the north. Indeed, only a few weeks before the trip, the government had indicted Kim Dae Jong, one of two principal leaders of the (majority) opposition parties in the National Assembly, for having accepted funds that originated in North Korea, and throughout the period the government put great pressure on those who sought to communicate with the north on their own. The official view of these moves to limit contact with the regime of North Korean leader Kim Il Sung was that the issue was one of law and order—South Korean law clearly outlaws any personal contact with the north—but it was, at heart, a political issue of great moment, and the indictment of Kim Dae Jong was seen by many as a harbinger of a return to the bad old days of authoritarian rule.

In the United States, however, Roh Tae Woo's stock was clearly on the rise. His moves toward democratization were both praised and encouraged by official Washington, and even the Korean position on trade with the United States—always a thorny issue—was being cast in a positive light. In the summer of 1989, the Koreans had—much to the amazement of persons close to the issue and to the envy of some other governments—escaped designation under so-called Super 301 legislation as deserving of U.S. trade sanctions. They accomplished this feat by sending a high-level delegation to Washington at the very last moment and making significant trade concessions, but also by drawing on some of their recently acquired political capital.

According to one official involved in planning the Roh visit, when President Bush visited Seoul briefly at the time of the funeral of Japanese Emperor Hirohito, he and Roh both expressed interest in a Washington visit by the Korean president. In July of 1989, Bush suggested that this take the form of an official working visit. It is clear that the Koreans would have preferred a state visit, but they agreed to working-visit status. While there is an ongoing, three-part agenda in U.S.-Korean relations—with discussion continuing over security issues, economic ties, and political structures—it appears that, in advance of the president's visit, the trip had few distinct policy objectives. Rather, it was intended primarily to show both the Korean and American publics that President Roh had good relations with the Bush administration. In effect, then, the visit—indeed, the *exchange* of visits initiated by Mr. Bush—was designed in large measure to symbolize the importance of the bilateral relationship. For all of its symbolic aspects, however, this objective does accord with a well-established substantive goal of Korean foreign policy, the desire to be accepted as a member of the community of industrialized nations. This same goal contributed significantly to the Korean decision to host the 1988 Olympic Games, which we will examine two chapters hence.

Planning for the visit involved coordination between Seoul and the embassy in Washington. Basic scheduling instructions were forwarded from the ministry of foreign affairs in Seoul to the first secretary for political affairs at the embassy in Washington, whose charge was to make them fit the circumstances in the United States. To accomplish this, the first secretary worked with an assistant chief of protocol at the State Department, clearing any decisions that were made with his superiors in Korea. In addition, the political affairs staff at the embassy would recommend, again through the first secretary, specific questions that the president might address during his trip. To handle the logistics of the visit—which included an entourage of some two hundred persons—the embassy staffers took on particular areas of responsibility. One staff member was responsible for all automobiles, one for hotels, one for all airplane and luggage arrangements, one for overseeing security, and so forth.

As the trip approached, Seoul provided limited guidance to the embassy in Washington as to what themes the government wanted to strike in its public, as opposed to its private, diplomacy. A delegation headed by the minister of state for legislative affairs (and later ambassador to the United States) Hyun Hong Choo spent a week in Washington during the month before the state visit, but left without addressing this question. The embassy view in the weeks before the visit was that the president should bring with him a clear message supporting democracy. This would be similar to the message conveyed some months earlier by Pakistani Prime Minister Benazir Bhutto with considerable effect.

The plans for the presidential visit were, in many ways, typical of the Korean approach to relations with the United States. Korean diplomacy, even public diplomacy, in general is addressed much more directly to American political elites than to the general public, a strategy that clearly suffused planning for the presidential visit. While the president's schedule called for a breakfast with Katherine Graham, publisher of the *Washington Post,* and with a number of journalists, a luncheon speech at the National Press Club, an address before a joint session of Congress, and a meeting with the World Affairs Council in Los Angeles, for example, no effort was made to set appearances on any of the several network news and public affairs broadcasts through which state visitors typically address the public more directly.

President Roh's objectives in advance of his visit were to present a ''correct'' (favorable) image of Korea to the U.S. public and to demonstrate to Koreans his ability to work on even terms with the American president. The first of these he intended to accomplish through a ''frank'' discussion with President Bush—recall that ''frank,'' the descriptor used by Korean sources beforehand to characterize the planned visit, is a term that, in diplomatic parlance, suggests the presence of significant disagreements between the parties—which would focus on means by which the two countries might lower the profile of the issues that divided them. Indeed, the Koreans took steps in that direction from the outset, having scheduled the press briefing on the president's visit, not in Washington where it might attract attention from the U.S. press, but in Seoul, where few American news agencies are permanently represented. No effort was made to ''hype'' the visit within the United States, except for a multipage insert on South Korea in the *Washington Post* of the type analyzed by Amaize and Faber (1983).

The second objective, that related to the domestic impact of the Roh visit, may have been the more important for the Korean president in the near term and the more difficult to achieve. According to Korean diplomats and journalists, the relationship between Korea and the United States was more routine at the time of the Roh trip than it had been in the recent past, and the visit itself was not seen as a "big deal." All the president had to do was to create the impression that he was well-treated and that Korea was important and respected in the United States. At the same time, however, the trip was not without its political risks. If Roh received no concessions from President Bush—and worse yet, if he made some of his own—he would be criticized by opposition forces at home for having been "scolded by Big Brother" and for having sold out Korea's national interests to the U.S. imperialists. That the Koreans did not rate this danger as very great is suggested by the fact that they did not schedule any special meetings during the visit with members of Congress who had been especially supportive of their recent political reforms, notably Representative Stephen Solarz and Senator Allan Cranston, with whom they maintained regular exchanges.

One typical add-on for a head-of-state visit is the awarding of an honorary degree to the visitor by an American university, though this is generally arranged outside of State Department channels. President Roh, for example, received such a degree from George Washington University. And here, too, we can see at work the same mix of communication strategy evident elsewhere in the visit, one that would yield minimal public exposure in the United States and an image of maximal international prestige at home. The awarding of the degree by GWU in particular was of special value to the president because that university is viewed in Korea as an especially prestigious one. This is attributable in large measure to the fact that Korea's first president, Singhman Rhee, attended GWU, and additionally to the (related) fact that many Korean business leaders today are graduates of the university. An honorary degree from that particular university thus had special value in a Korean context, and the award ceremony was covered extensively by Korean journalists, including camera crews from both television networks. At the same time, the ceremony was held at the official residence of the Korean ambassador in Washington and was open by invitation only. No American reporters were present (other than the editor of the university's student newspaper), and the event received no coverage at all in the American press.

Indeed, the entire visit attracted relatively little media attention in the United States—the *New York Times,* for example, published only one story on the subject—and the level of news coverage of Korea overall in the aftermath of the visit remained minimal. This lowering of the volume was clearly in line with Korean public diplomacy objectives. Unfortunately, however, the coverage that was accorded did not cast Korean-American relations in as favorable a light as the Koreans might have hoped. The essence of the *Times* story on the presidential visit, for example, is captured in the associated entry in the *Times Index:* "Pres Roh Tae Woo of South Korea, addressing joint meeting of Congress in Washington, seeks to assure Congress that anti-Americanism in his country is limited to handful of radicals; also urges United States not to cut 43,000 American troops in South Korea." (Compare this with the summary of Bhutto's address cited in Chapter 5.) The net result, then, was probably not an improvement in Korea's image among the American media and public. And the substantive payoff of the visit? In January 1990, after what might be considered a decent diplomatic interval, the two governments announced an agreement to reduce the number of U.S. troops in South Korea, and in February a Korean official told the *Times* that the withdrawals would amount to more than the minor reduction implied in January.

The Medium Is the Message

In their official travel, foreign heads of state and government do not, by and large, come to the United States as tourists, and it is not the monuments and museums of the nation's capital that draw them to Washington. They come to the United States to gain political advantage, sometimes in their respective domestic spheres and sometimes internationally. They come to Washington because it is, for them, the center of American political and media power and because they want some of the benefits that power can bestow.

For all of that, however, foreign leaders come to the United States under diverse circumstances—some of their own making and some of American or other manufacture—and with the widely differing menus of needs those diverse circumstances generate. Typically, when public or scholarly attention focuses on visits by foreign leaders, it does so by looking at policy objectives and accomplishments. What did Churchill, Roosevelt, and Stalin accomplish at Potsdam? What did Reagan and Gorbachev really agree to in Reykjavik? It is the objective of the present research, however, to point out that the accomplishments of government-to-government diplomacy are neither automatic nor focused exclusively on expressly foreign *policy* outcomes. Rather, these visits achieve (or fail to achieve) their policy objectives in some considerable measure because of the communication planning that precedes, accompanies, and even follows them. And their objectives may often include specific public diplomacy goals. This was clearly the case in the visit examined here—with the Koreans seeking to lower the temperature of their relations with the United States—and was the case as well when Pakistani Prime Minister Benazir Bhutto came to Washington in the same year, to be discussed in Chapter 5, though in that instance the prime minister's intention was in part to raise visibility rather than to lower it. Both leaders had an agenda of substantive policy objectives, and both saw the need to manage media portrayals of their respective visits. Communication strategies, in other words, are important means through which the goals of statecraft can be accomplished.

Moreover, the decisions as to how to accomplish these public diplomacy objectives, and the ability to implement them, are neither uniform nor automatic. At both the strategic and the tactical levels, they require an understanding of the potential audience for the visiting leader's message and of significant segments thereof, a command of the appropriate channels for reaching the target audience and avoiding eavesdroppers (and an understanding of the differentiation among channels), the generation of the "right" message to accomplish the public diplomacy or policy objectives, and a modicum of communication skill. All of these elements represent variables that are worthy of scholarly attention. Collectively, and in combination with the communication setting, they produce outcomes that can, quite literally, shake the world—or at least significant corners of it.

5

What's in a Word?: "Democracy" and U.S. Foreign Policy

[Democracy is] the sense of spiritual independence which nerves the individual to stand alone against the powers of the world.
RICHARD H. TAWNEY

[Democracy is] the fairest of names, but the worst of realities—mob rule.
POLYBIUS

We believe that our democracy in China is the best democracy. When the young students in China talked about their understanding of democracy and freedom last year, what they aspired to was freedom or democracy that cannot be found in this world . . . . We do not regret, or criticize ourselves for the way we handled, the Tiananmen event, because if we had not sent in the troops I would not be able to sit here today.
JIANG ZEMIN, General Secretary, Chinese Communist Party

[Democracy] has come to mean whatever anyone wants it to mean.
BERNARD SMITH

Our review of the agencies and decisions involved in planning state visits to Washington, as illustrated by the 1989 visit of Korean President Roh Tae Woo, provides us with a baseline for understanding the core motivations and mechanisms by which everyday public diplomacy is conducted. In this chapter, we will take a look at how this routine process can be transformed at the hands of a strategic communications consultant from an occasion for diplomatic exchange into a campaign for the hearts and minds of the American people, or at least for key members of their political leadership.

Partners in Democracy

Benazir Bhutto is the daughter of the late Pakistani President Zulfikar Ali Bhutto, who was hanged after a lengthy imprisonment by his successor, General Zia Ul Haq. General Zia was himself the victim of suspected foul play, having been killed in a 1988 plane crash that also took the life of the American ambassador to Pakistan. Following an intensely competitive election campaign after Zia's death and a period of intense negotiation with his former supporters, Benazir Bhutto was named prime minister of Pakistan.

As prime minister, Bhutto confronted a wide range of problems including the need to control and repatriate tens of thousands of Afghan refugees and to consolidate some support—or at least to demobilize any potential opposition—among the Pakistani military. In many ways, the United States held the key to her ability to meet these challenges. But following the Soviet withdrawal from Afghanistan in February 1989, American interest in Pakistan evidenced a marked decline. In an effort to restore that interest and to obtain assistance that was vital to her political—and perhaps her personal—survival, Bhutto arranged a visit to the United States in June 1989. It is that visit—and more particularly its strong component of strategic communication—that provides our focus of attention here.

To assist in the planning of her visit, Bhutto hired American lobbyist and political consultant Mark Siegel. Though he eschews the title, Siegel is a good example of the new generation of strategic communication professionals. He received his doctoral degree in political science from Northwestern University in 1972 and, after a brief stint in teaching, moved to Washington, where he became executive director of the Democratic National Committee. He later served in the Carter White House and worked on contract for AIPAC, the American-Israel Political Action Committee, before forming his own lobbying and consulting firm, Mark A. Siegel and Associates. Though most of his clientele was domestic, he did serve some foreign interests such as the government of Aruba. Siegel had known Benazir Bhutto since her days at Harvard and had, for some time, provided political advice to her and her political party. When she became prime minister, Bhutto signed a $400,000 contract with Siegel—who formed a separate company, International Public Strategies, Inc., principally to service this new account—to provide advice to, and representation in behalf of, her government. One of Siegel's first responsibilities was to plan her first official visit to Washington.

Siegel approached the Bhutto visit as if it were a domestic political campaign, albeit one limited to less than a week. Given the prime minister's need to raise the visibility of her country in foreign policy dialogue within the United States, he determined that Bhutto should attempt to dominate the media for the four to five days of her visit, and that all of her appearances should have one unifying theme so that they appeared to be parts of a single, and very important, event. The U.S. government cooperated in assuring a high-visibility trip by classifying it as an official visit, with the higher order of pomp and circumstance, and of presidential participation, that that designation entailed.

In much the same way that a campaign consultant manages access to a candidate, Siegel managed access to Bhutto. In advance of the visit, he negotiated appearances on the *MacNeil/Lehrer NewsHour* (PBS) and *60 Minutes* (CBS), as well as an interview with Connie Chung (at the time with NBC). And once the prime minister arrived in the United States, Siegel made careful efforts to control which journalists gained access to her—not because he was concerned over Bhutto's ability to deal with the American media, which, in fact, he saw as one of her major strengths, but because he wanted to expose her only to journalists who might be expected to ask the most sophisticated questions and to address the central issues of Pakistani-American relations rather than lesser topics (e.g., of the woman-leading-government type) that Siegel regarded as "distractions." Such questioning by premier journalists, he thought, would enhance her prestige simply by association, while her answers would provide additional opportunities to promote the theme of the visit. Siegel worked closely with the staffs of NBC and ABC News to prepare for Bhutto's *Today* and Peter Jennings interviews during the visit.

The theme that was adopted for the Bhutto visit was that of a democratic partnership with new priorities, and all of the "campaign" activities reinforced this message. The centerpiece of the visit was Bhutto's address at the Harvard University commencement, where she called for the creation of an association of democratic nations, one in which the richest democracies would aid the poorest and through which economic and political sanctions might be applied against those nations moving away from the democratic ideal. The United States, as the world's oldest democracy, she suggested, and Pakistan, at the time its newest, should work together to bring such an association into being. Developing the same theme in her address to a joint session of Congress—which Siegel was able to arrange because of his contacts within the Democratic leadership—she sought to reinforce her strategic base of political support among American conservatives, while broadening it to include some political liberals.

The consistency with which this theme was pursued is evident from a sampling of Bhutto's rhetoric during her visit (emphasis added in each instance). In sequential order:

- To President Bush at the White House arrival ceremony: "Our two nations now bonded in *democracy,* bonded in common goals and common interests, bonded together in our commitment to freedom and liberty."

- To Vice President Quayle in a toast: "The United States and Pakistan are bonded together based on trust, on common interest, on common goals, and now, at long last, on a common, democratic form of government. . . . We come here, the world's newest *democracy* to the world's greatest *democracy,* in friendship, in partnership, in good will."

- To the Congress of the United States: "America's greatest contribution to the world is its concept of *democracy,* its concept of freedom, freedom of action, freedom of speech, and freedom of thought. . . . For decades we have been tied together by mutual international goals, and by shared interests. But something new has entered into the equation of bilateral relations—*democracy*. We are now moral as well as political partners."

- To the audience at Harvard's commencement, where she was the featured speaker: "Democratic nations should forge a consensus around the most powerful political idea in the world today: the right of people to freely choose their government. Having created a bond through evolving such a consensus, democratic nations should then come together in an association to help each other and promote what is a universal value—*democracy.*"

- To Senator Edward Kennedy in a ceremony at the Kennedy Presidential Library: ". . . the Bhutto family feels a unique kinship with your family. It is a kinship that comes from a common commitment to . . . *democracy* and human rights. . . ."

- To the Annual Meeting of The Asia Society: "And it is Asia today where *democracy* is being reborn amid the ashes of dictatorship. My presence here this evening is a testament to the force of *democracy* in Pakistan. . . . Freedom is not an end. Freedom is just the beginning. And in Pakistan, at long last, we are ready to begin."

Altogether, as Table 5.1 shows, the words "democrat," "democracy," "democratic," and others with the same root occured a total of 103 times in the official texts of these six speeches and statements—all of which were drafted by Siegel and his staff—or roughly 3.5 times per page. In none of these statements were there fewer than 5 such references, while the Harvard address contained fully *51*. On average, then, the prime minister was uttering one of these words more than once per minute throughout her public appearances in the United States. These were liberally supplemented by frequent references to freedom, liberty, and constitutional government and seasoned with quotations from Americans historically associated with democratic values, most notably James Madison and Abraham Lincoln. In addition, International Public Strategies issued a position paper supporting the centerpiece of Bhutto's Harvard speech, a call for establishing an Association of Democratic Nations. In seven pages of text, this document managed to incorporate 59 references to democracy, or more than 8 per page.

Still following the campaign analogy, Siegel viewed the joint session and Harvard appearances as "paid media" and the several interviews the prime minister granted in advance of and during her trip as "free media." The paid-media messages were carefully crafted with attention to thematic consistency and were presented under tightly controlled conditions to a preselected primary audience—the Harvard commencement, with its tradition of forward-looking proposals from prominent leaders, for the intellectual substance and spiritual guidance of the message and the joint session for the political context. The free-media messages were channeled insofar as possible to settings and journalists who—by doing their jobs in precisely the ways they otherwise would—would serve the prime minister's needs.

What did Bhutto and Pakistan accomplish through this effort? She did play to rave reviews in the *New York Times*. One entry in the *Times*

Table 5.1. References to Democracy and Related Words in Public Statements of Prime Minister Benazir Bhutto of Pakistan During Official Visit to United States: June 1989

Statement	Est. No. of Words	Democracy References	Freedom References	Liberty/ Justice References	Elective Status References
White House	300	5	4	1	2
Vice President Toast	300	7	1	0	0
Joint Session	1,600	22	25	2	4
Harvard	2,000	51	17	8	12
Kennedy Library	400	6	1	1	1
Asia Society	1,400	12	6	1	1
Total	6,000	103	54	13	20

Index seems to capture the spirit in which the newspaper viewed her visit. "Prime Minister Benazir Bhutto of Pakistan," it stated, "addresses joint meeting of Congress in Washington, captivating it with speech that portrays herself as embodiment of democracy, spokesman for women, youth, and those in Islamic mainstream, fighter for freedom in Afghanistan and political descendant of John F. Kennedy." In contrast, recall the index entry that followed President Roh's address to the same body. On the other hand, as we will see, the coverage of Pakistan in the *Washington Post* did not reflect any systematic increase in references to the democracy theme during the months immediately following Bhutto's visit. In June, for example, the month of the visit, the *Post* carried only one article on Pakistani political affairs and no references to the democracy theme occurred following the visit until October and November, when there was a brief flurry of attention to this topic.[1]

Another locus of possible effects of the visit and its central emphasis may be found in the level of Pakistan-related activity among politicians and journalists in Washington during the periods just before, during, and just after the prime minister's visit. To assess the importance and character of Pakistan's place on the agenda of American opinion makers in each of these time periods, I employed the *Legi-Slate* database. Included in the database were selected transcripts of committee hearings from the House and Senate; news briefings from the White House and six cabinet departments; speeches, news conferences, and interviews by the president, cabinet secretaries, other administration officials, visiting heads of state, and other dignitaries; and television public affairs programs including the principal Sunday programs (e.g., *Meet the Press*), the network morning programs, CNN's major news interviews, and USIA's *Worldnet*.[2]

The prime minister's visit began officially June 6, though she actually arrived in Washington the day before. To assess the effect of the visit, I searched all transcripts from all sources except the Department of Defense for the period May 1 through July 31, 1990, for any that included a reference to Pakistan. This search identified fifty-eight transcripts. Of these, seventeen occurred between May 1 and June 4, nineteen between June 5 and June 9, the period of Bhutto's visit, and the balance between June 10 and the end of July. During the first of these periods, congressional hearings dominated the transcripts; in the second period, as one might expect, media coverage and official statements predominated; and the final period included a mix primarily of congressional hearings and press briefings.

Though it is difficult to quantify, the difference in tone between previsit and postvisit transcripts is quite notable. This may best be captured in a brief selection of comments from each period.

Before the visit:

- Testimony before a Senate Governmental Affairs Committee hearing on chemical and biological weapons: "We're seeing continued efforts by would-be proliferators to acquire basic materials and technology . . . using . . . many of the same type of shady procurement techniques that Pakistan has been using to acquire materials for its nuclear weapon program."
- David Westgate, Director of Drug Enforcement Operations, DEA, in a speech at the National Press Club: "Most of this is Southeast Asian heroin, which is a change from Southwest Asian—Southwest being Pakistan. . . ."
- Roberto Eisenmann, former editor of *La Prensa,* in a speech at the National Press Club: "We saw it in Pakistan; we saw it in Greece; we saw it in Argentina; Idi Amin in Uganda; Bocasa in Central Africa. It's normal for these regimes, when they get to the point where they have no political base, to look for an external enemy to try and justify their existence. . . ."
- William Webster, Director of the CIA, testifying before the Senate

Governmental Affairs Committee on the subject of nuclear prolif-
eration: "I think that for [India and Pakistan] to develop, to be
dedicating so much of their resources in this area, is a cause for
international concern about stability in the region.

During this period, only one speaker, Ambassador Max Kampelman,
made any substantive positive reference to Pakistan. In a speech at the
Jamestown Foundation Awards Dinner, he linked Pakistan with South
Korea, the Philippines, South Africa, China, Poland, and other countries where he saw people living in greater freedom than in the past.
"This trend is prompted," said Kampelman, "not only by an abstract
love of justice . . . but by the growing realization that democracy
works best." This comment notwithstanding, however, the overwhelming proportion of references to Pakistan in advance of the Bhutto visit
were unfavorable.

After the visit:

- Senator Gordon Humphrey, at a hearing of the Asian and Pacific
  Affairs Subcommittee of the House Foreign Affairs Committee:
  "Just last week the prime minister of Pakistan, in her impressive
  address to the joint session, reminded us that our objective has been
  self-determination for the people of Afghanistan. And the prime
  minister pointed out that for ten years the United States has stood
  side by side with Pakistan. . . ."
- Ambassador Howard Shaffer, at a subsequent session of the same
  subcommittee: "Pakistan's commitment to peace and democracy
  are [*sic*] fundamental."
- Reza Pahlavi, son of the late shah of Iran, on CNN's *Newsmaker
  Sunday:* "I believe that when we look at the scenarios such as the
  one in Pakistan or in the Philippines, the democratic wave is starting in the whole world around. . . ."
- Australian Prime Minister Robert Hawke at a press conference:
  "[Indian Prime Minister Rajiv Gandhi] told me that he had established a good, he thought, friendly, constructive relation with
  Prime Minister Benazir Bhutto of Pakistan, and particularly
  thought that after the next Indian elections . . . there was the opportunity for a constructive resolution of their border problems."
- President Bush in a statement at the White House ceremony for
  Captive Nations Week: "We see that truth in the successful return
  of democracy to Pakistan. . . ."

The period closed with an extensive interview of Bhutto on CNN's *International Hour,* where the prime minister was introduced as having returned from exile "to win Pakistan's first democratic election in more than a decade." Collectively, then, these and other references during the roughly seven weeks following Bhutto's visit portrayed Pakistan in a much more favorable light than had been the case previously.

Ultimately, however, the measure of success most vital to Bhutto lay in her ability to coax from Washington the movement in American foreign policy that she required. Here, too, there were substantial gains. Annual aid to Pakistan was increased $50 million to $680 million at a time when most foreign aid awards were shrinking; after what had been a lengthy delay, final approval was given for the sale to Pakistan of sixty advanced F-16 fighter aircraft, a deal valued at $1.5 billion; and—especially noteworthy, perhaps, in light of the very public concern of the U.S. government over nuclear proliferation during the previsit period—the United States dropped its demand that Pakistan pledge not to enrich uranium beyond 5 percent.

What's the Good Word?

There are many factors that can help to explain Prime Minister Bhutto's success during her 1989 state visit. Bhutto herself was viewed favorably in official Washington, where she was seen as a force for modernization in Pakistan, and in the wake of the Afghan civil war, the United States was open to a new hook on which to hang its policy toward South Asia. Moreover, commitments had been made to Pakistan that had not been fulfilled. But none of these factors made inevitable the turn toward Pakistan that the Bhutto visit produced. Indeed, one might argue that similar preconditions provided context for the Roh Tae Woo visit, yet the Korean president left town with far less in his pocket.

What made the Bhutto visit so successful, I believe, was the fact that she was able to recognize and take full advantage of the favorable environment surrounding the visit. In that, Mark Siegel's campaign played a significant role. And the key to Siegel's effort lay in a single word, which is, of course, obvious by now: democracy. If Siegel could create an equation in the minds of the American public, the media, and the political elite—Bhutto = democracy—he knew he could carry the day. He understood this for two reasons, one theoretical and one political.

At the theoretical level, what Siegel and others like him attempt to do for their clients is to "frame" public perceptions by associating the client leader or country with established and highly regarded values that are already present in the public mind. They do this by providing what students of the process term "cues," words or visual images that tie the client to the target value. To the extent that these cues dominate portrayals of the client in the media or other public discourse, and to the extent that they do not conflict with other client-related images that might already be in place, they have the potential to shape (frame) perceptions, and through them, the policy environment, at the least creating opportunities for advantage and at best creating positive momentum in the desired direction.[3]

As John Zaller (1992) has shown, it is particularly important to shape the discourse of the members of the policy elite because they, in turn, will frame issues for the media and the most attentive segments of the general public. We saw a good example of this phenomenon in the mobilization of support for the Gulf War, in which the degree of legitimacy accorded by the media to opposition to military action and the range of acceptable debate expanded and contracted depending on the views expressed by so-called "official" voices. When members of the elite engaged in wide-ranging debate, the range of views expressed in and by the media broadened. When the official consensus was more focused, so, too, was the media consensus (Bennett and Manheim, 1993).

Mark Siegel's emphasis on setting the terms of elite debate over American policy toward Pakistan, then, was well justified. And his emphasis on democracy, per se, was equally on target. Americans have long regarded themselves as the keepers of the democratic flame, and many of their most significant foreign policy undertakings have been rationalized for domestic purposes as prodemocracy initiatives. Never was this sense of democratic self more resonant than at the very time of the Bhutto visit in June 1989. Therein lies the link between theoretical constructs and political realities.

In the spring of 1989, just weeks before the Bhutto visit, thousands of young Chinese demonstrators had occupied Tiananmen Square in the political heart of Beijing. But the images from Tiananmen Square—of a lone man halting a column of tanks, of styrofoam sculptures of the Statue of Liberty and the Goddess of Democracy, of a chorus of "We Shall Overcome"—were aimed straight at the political heart—or at least the heart*strings*—of a nation an ocean away. For, their evident domestic significance notwithstanding, many of these actions were also staged for the benefit of foreign—notably American—audiences. The demonstrations that developed into the Beijing Spring, after all, were timed to coincide with the arrival in the Chinese capital of Mikhail Gorbachev for the first top-level Sino-Soviet exchange in decades, and an event that, at the time, was still regarded as significant. This strategy provided increased leverage on the Chinese leadership, in no small measure because it guaranteed the presence of the world press. Similarly, the foam model of the Statue of Liberty created an extraordinary "photo opportunity," albeit one whose roots in *Chinese* culture would be difficult to trace. The anthem of the American civil rights movement has gained world popularity, but it is not always sung—as it was in Tiananmen—in English. And, too, many of the banners and signs around the square were printed in English. The signs of a consistent strategy of appealing to foreign publics—and expressly to the American public—were manifold.[4]

This observation is all the more interesting when one considers the objectives of the demonstrators and how those objectives were transformed during the early days of the Tiananmen occupation. First reports from the scene suggested that what the Chinese students really wanted was "democratic" reform *within the Chinese Communist Party*. Indeed, some early commentaries suggested that many of the students were about to enter the Chinese version of the job market and that their principal objective was to end the system of favoritism under which the best positions went to the children of the political elite. These were not objectives with which many Americans or other foreigners might be expected to identify—at least at an emotional level—but they were apparently the initial goals of many demonstrators. It was only later, as media coverage developed and the occupation of the square and confrontation with the government grew, that broader objectives were conveyed and that "democracy" in some larger sense became the driving force of the action.

While the events in Tiananmen Square in 1989 have their own significance, both for Chinese politics and American, it is our vivid recall of the words and images of Beijing Spring that is most germane to the present argument. For in the vividness of that recall is prima facie evidence of the potency of "democracy" as a symbol in public diplomacy. By referencing democracy—and in particular *American* democracy—the students of Tiananmen struck a chord in the American people—at least most of them—that resonates to this day. Their degree of success in employing symbols of democracy may have been unusual, but their selection of democratic cues per se was not.

Indeed, though it is interesting to examine cases like the Bhutto visit or the Tiananmen demonstrations and extract from them lessons regarding the framing of perceptions and their effect on the making of U.S. foreign policy, these examples suffer all the shortcomings of the case-study approach. Most notably, they are of limited generalizability. Each may have idiosyncratic elements that prevents our drawing broadly applicable conclusions from our observations. To remedy that, we will conclude the present chapter with a more expressly quantitative examination of one aspect of the same question we have addressed anecdotally here: To what extent do images of "democracy" shape American perceptions and discourse regarding different regions and nations of the world?

Media and "Democracy"

Specifically, we will examine the frequency and distribution of references to democracy in the news media. To test for the presence of such cues in news of foreign affairs, I examined the coverage of political affairs in some twenty countries carried in the electronic version of the *Washington Post* during the period March 1985 through May 1990.[5] The electronic *Post* was accessed through the *Legi-Slate* database. It comprises approximately seventy-five articles per day that are judged by the editors of the newspaper itself (*Legi-Slate* is a subsidiary of The Washington Post Company) as most significant. A search of the database by country identified roughly 25,000 insertions about the target countries during the five and one-quarter years for which data were available at the time of this study.[6] From these articles, I selected a subset that had been coded by *Legi-Slate* as pertaining to political affairs. This procedure yielded 6,614 insertions, each of which was then scanned electronically for the presence of the word "democracy." The results were compiled into monthly summaries which provide the basis for the analysis that follows.

Table 5.2 summarizes the findings of this analysis grouped by region for four areas: Eastern Europe, Africa, Latin America, and Asia. The table reports seven indicators:

Table 5.2. Political Affairs Coverage in the *Washington Post*, Aggregates and Monthly Averages by Region: March 1985–May 1990

Region	No. of Insertions	No. of Political Affairs Insertions	No. of Democracy Insertions	Mean Insertions	Mean Political Affairs Insertions	Mean Democracy Insertions	% Political Affairs w/ Democracy References
Eastern Europe	4,259	1,667	612	67.6	26.5	9.7	37
Africa	4,726	1,235	166	75.0	19.6	2.6	13
Latin America	7,927	1,671	403	125.8	26.5	6.4	24
Asia	7,906	2,041	754	125.5	32.4	12.0	37
Total	24,818	6,614	1,935	393.9	105.0	30.7	29

- the total number of insertions (news items, editorials, etc.) about the five selected countries within each region published in the *Post* during the study period;
- the number of these insertions that dealt with political affairs;
- the number of political affairs insertions that included at least one mention of the word "democracy";
- the monthly averages of each of the preceeding indicators; and
- the percentage of all political affairs insertions that included "democracy" references.

Of particular interest are the last two listed indicators, the average number of "democracy" references and the proportion of insertions in which they occur.

The table shows a rather clear pattern of differentiation in the use of "democracy" references. In absolute terms, as measured by the average number of references per month, the democracy theme has been applied most extensively to Asian countries, with Eastern Europe following close behind. Latin America is a distant third, and Africa trails. When we control for the fact that different regions of the world receive differing amounts of overall coverage—a fact that is itself quite interesting but lies beyond the scope of the present analysis—by looking at the percentage of articles with references to democracy (column seven) rather than at the total number of such references, we find that democracy is a theme in more than a third of the stories on both Asia and Eastern Europe—a remarkably high percentage given our criterion that each insertion must contain the specific word "democracy"—but in barely a tenth of those on Africa. In effect, then, the newspaper is conveying the message to its readers that "the story" in Asia and Eastern Europe is a story of democracy, while in Latin America and Africa it is something else. Put another way, readers of the *Washington Post* during this period were being prepared to view events in Asia and Eastern Europe as components of a struggle for democratic progress, a news frame that was not applied even to Latin American and African countries, which under the selection criteria employed in this research, could have made similar claims to democratization. In those regions, some other news frame was being employed and another message conveyed.

To determine what that alternative news frame might be, I conducted a similar analysis on the same selection of articles using alternative terms. With respect to Latin America, the news employed a mix of cues, but fully 290 insertions, or 17 percent of the total, included a reference to drug-related activity. News of Africa was dominated by coverage of events relating to South Africa. Some 448 stories, or 36 percent (nearly three times the rate for democracy) included the term "apartheid," while 300 insertions, or 24 percent of the total, included the phrase "African National Congress." Each of these ancillary findings makes intuitive sense, and that is, perhaps, the very point. In Colombia, for example, much of the contemporaneous struggle between the government and the drug lords could readily have been characterized as a struggle for the survival of democratic institutions, while in South Africa the movement toward majority rule could readily have been portrayed as the evolution of such institutions. What the evidence shows, however, is that, during that five-year period, the media, or at least the editors of the *Washington Post,* chose systematically to portray these events in other terms.

The consistency of these decisions becomes more apparent when we examine Table 5.3, which reports the same data broken out by each component country. Of the original seven indicators, perhaps the most interesting here is that summarizing the percentage of each country's political affairs coverage that includes a democracy reference. In Asia, that percentage ranged from 28 to 57 and in Eastern Europe from 32 to 49 percent. By comparison, Latin American countries score between 20 and 31 percent on the indicator and African countries between 7 and 21. There is, in short, relatively little variation evident around the respective regional means, which suggests that the *Post* editors paint with a broad brush.

Adding dimension to the analysis of Table 5.3 is an eighth indicator, which I have labeled "focus." Given the rather lengthy period covered by this study, more than five years, two patterns of democratic references might emerge at the extremes. On the one hand, references to democracy might be recurrent elements of a country's news portrayal throughout the period. Such references might aggregate over time to a sizeable number, but might nevertheless occur in such small numbers at any given time that they fail to impact significantly on the public's consciousness. On the other hand, where references to democracy (or any other theme) are intensively concentrated during a relatively short time period, and where the country in question is featured prominently in the news, such cues can be expected to define the story.

Reported under "focus" is the minimum number of months at any

Table 5.3. Political Affairs Coverage in the *Washington Post*, Aggregates and Monthly Averages by Country: March 1985–May 1990

Country	No. of Inserts	No. of Political Affairs Inserts	No. of Democracy Inserts	Mean Inserts	Mean Political Affairs Inserts	Mean Democracy Inserts	% Political Affairs w/ Democracy	Focus
			Eastern Europe					
Albania	99	49	17	1.6	0.8	0.3	35	4
Bulgaria	411	142	69	6.5	2.3	1.1	49	3
Czechoslovakia	1,049	427	168	16.7	6.8	2.7	39	4
Poland	2,101	822	261	33.3	13.0	4.1	32	6
Romania	599	227	97	9.5	3.6	1.5	43	3
			Africa					
Angola	777	156	21	12.3	2.5	0.3	13	8
Mozambique	306	71	5	4.9	1.1	0.1	7	14
Namibia	429	102	21	6.8	1.6	0.3	21	7
South Africa	2,848	834	105	45.2	13.2	1.7	13	22
Sudan	366	72	14	5.8	1.1	0.2	19	15

Latin America

Bolivia	307	39	12	4.9	0.6	0.2	31	26
Colombia	915	159	32	14.5	2.5	0.5	20	8
Mexico	1,843	280	65	29.3	4.4	1.0	23	19
Nicaragua	4,294	1080	265	68.2	17.1	4.2	25	29
Peru	568	113	29	9.0	1.8	0.5	26	16

Asia

China	3,146	828	360	49.9	13.1	5.7	43	8
Nepal	73	21	12	1.2	0.3	0.2	57	2
Pakistan	1,256	268	75	19.9	4.3	1.2	28	22
Philippines	1,645	494	148	26.1	7.8	2.3	30	16
South Korea	1,786	430	159	28.3	6.8	2.5	37	13

point in the series of observations for each country that was required to account for at least fifty percent of all references to "democracy." Thus, the higher this number, the more diffuse the references and the less likely they would have been to frame public perceptions of the country, and the lower the number, the more concentrated and, probably, the more effective the framing. Here we do find some significant concentration in at least one country of each region, but with only one exception—Nepal, where almost the only coverage of the entire period centered on the reform movement of 1990—all of the lowest values (greatest concentrations) occured in Eastern Europe.

Combining these measures of intensity with our observations on the overall news visibility of each country, what we see is that "democracy" was the dominant news frame—the defining element of the story—in Eastern Europe and China, even in Romania with its apparent coup d'état and in Bulgaria where the Communist elite was returned to power under a different label. But this was not the case in South Africa, nor in Nicaragua, and not nearly so much in the Philippines or South Korea, to name but a few. Yet, *if* one accepts the argument that events in each of these countries resembled one another in that they represented movement toward political systems that were either genuinely or apparently more democratic—and that is, admittedly, a big lump to swallow—then one might reasonably expect, other things being equal, that the portrayal of each country in the press would resemble that of the others more or less closely. That this is clearly not the case suggests that the *ceteris* are not *paribus*. Other things are not equal.

The reasons why story lines might vary across countries and regions are manifold—they trace to the full panoply of newsroom decision making described, for example, by Bennett (1988)—and lie, for the most part, beyond the scope of the present inquiry. One such reason, however, has been hinted already and does deserve our direct attention. The hint came in our discussions of the staging of events both for the Bhutto visit and in Tiananmen Square, and the reason it reveals is the purposeful managing of the news through the various techniques of public diplomacy. In particular, the reason that some countries may be linked in the press to democratic themes is that they—or, as in the case of China, some significant albeit unofficial persons or groups in them—set about more or less purposefully to encourage precisely such a linkage.

Conclusion

We began this chapter with a look at a systematic campaign to establish in the political discourse of the United States an image of Benazir Bhutto and Pakistan as partners in democracy and concluded with a more general analysis of the distribution of this democratic frame of reference among diverse countries and regions. From the evidence provided, three arguments should begin to emerge. First, particular cues do, in fact, tend to be associated systematically with particular objects of foreign policy—governments, mass movements, individual leaders, and the like—at least in the news media. In even the limited analysis of articles in the *Washington Post* presented here, such patterns are quite evident. Second, a context of favorable cues creates a political environment in the United States that is relatively more supportive of a given country or leader than it would otherwise be. This requires a bit more of a leap of faith, but is supported in the extant case by the achievement of the policy objectives that had been set by Prime Minister Bhutto as well as by similar gains noted elsewhere in this volume. And third, foreign leaders and others are cognizant of this phenomenon and do, at least in certain instances, work to create precisely this kind of supportive symbolic environment in which to pursue their foreign policy objectives. In the next chapter, we will see just how far some countries will go to create a desired image and just how much trouble some of these efforts can cause them.

6

Rites of Passage: Mega-Events
as Public Diplomacy

The emphasis placed by many governments on head-of-state visits as foci of public diplomacy suggests the importance that defining events can play in communication strategy. But head-of-state visits are not the only types of events that can be employed for this purpose. Indeed, by some standards, they are relatively insignificant, especially when a government has the opportunity to parade its virtues before the entire world. In this chapter, we will focus on the utility of such global events as a component of a country's public diplomacy by examining one of the common forms, the staging of sporting spectacles. Our analysis will center on the hosting of the 1988 Summer Olympics by the Republic of Korea. One lesson we will learn is that even the most carefully planned of events can sometimes have unintended consequences.

Scholars in the tradition of Murray Edelman (e.g., 1988) see all of politics as a social construction or, in Edelman's term, a "spectacle," in which reality is a composite of the perceptions of those who experience or observe it. In such a world, the power to control perception is the power to control reality. And that control is exercised by those who are able to maintain authorship of key aspects of the human experience— those who interpret the drama of everyday political life (Combs, 1980).

Once we accept this notion, it is a short step to the realization that "political" is itself a term that is subject to widely varying interpretation. Elections are political, and wars are political.[1] But so, too, are other aspects of the life experience that seem at first view to be far removed. Because of its melodramatic potential and its immense audience appeal, sport is one such phenomenon (Nimmo and Combs, 1983).

Sport is the stuff of news. Considered in the light of what the literature tells us are the principal criteria of newsworthiness—drama, prominent actors, timeliness, conflict, accessibility, audience appeal (Bennett, 1988a)—it is little wonder that more media space/time and more audience attention are devoted to sports coverage than to international or even domestic political events in the U.S. media. Nor are politicians unaware of the draw of sport. From the local official who throws out the first baseball on opening day to the "ping-pong diplomacy" of major-power relations, political leaders commonly seek to use to their advantage the appeal of sport. And, because it holds the attention of large numbers of people in multiple countries and conveys to them simple and highly symbolic messages, high-level international sporting competition is inextricably linked with international politics. With their visible nationalistic elements (flags, uniforms) and the opportunities they provide propagandists and commentators alike to interpret individual or team accomplishments as tests of national character, will, and achievement, such sporting events provide a showcase for leaders or advocates of causes who compete for world attention (Hoberman, 1984: 7–1).

As Hazan (1982: 18) has put it:

> Sport . . . is a medium that may simultaneously embrace billions of people, an unsuspecting audience whose absorption screen is exposed and vulnerable and whose mental defenses against propaganda are completely down. It is a means of . . . penetrating all defenses, engaging the audience emotionally, vocally, and physically.

No international competition is more subject to such politicization than the quadrennial world's fair that is the Olympic Games (Taylor, 1986). Though the classical games were intended as a respite from politics, the modern games, with their boycotts and blacklists, their terrorist threats, and even their medal counts, are anything but. The 1936 Berlin games (described in Hart-Davis, 1986, and Mandell, 1987, and memorialized in the films of Leni Riefenstahl) established the genre, and the cold war tensions of Melbourne and Squaw Valley (Espy, 1979: 39–76), the violence of Münich, and the tit-for-tat politics of Moscow (Booker, 1981; Hazan, 1982; Hoberman, 1986) and Los Angeles ensured its endurance. It should come as no surprise, then, that in bidding in 1981 to host the summer games of 1988, the Korean government headed by

President Chun Doo Hwan had in mind a variety of economic and political objectives. Let us place those objectives in context by reviewing briefly the situation in South Korea at that time.

The Decision to Host the 1988 Summer Olympics

At its inception in 1980, the administration of President Chun confronted three prominent facts of political and economic life. First, the Korean economy was expanding rapidly. This was producing some social dislocation as the labor force shifted from a largely agrarian to a predominantly industrial economy and was beginning to produce a higher standard of living for substantial numbers of Koreans. Second, though the rising economic tide was starting to generate an accompanying set of rising political expectations, there was no general consensus on what precise form the Korean political system should take. There was, however, widespread unwillingness, especially among the younger generation and in certain regions of the country, to accept the legitimacy of the new government. This crisis of legitimacy was based in part on a general distrust of the continuing series of authoritarian military regimes, and in no small measure in reaction to the violence at Kwangju and its role as the crucible in which this latest amalgam was created. In a country where politics, even robustly democratic politics, is a rough-and-tumble game, the disadvantage to the government of allowing such opposition to fester unchecked was clear. Third, the North Korean regime continued a series of hostile acts (subsequently manifested in the assassination of several South Korean officials in Burma, and then in a bomb attack on a Korean Air flight) that highlighted the division of historic Korea at the thirty-eighth parallel. Each of these factors contributed to the government's decision to bid for the Olympics.

Foremost in this decision was the desire to call world attention to, and, not incidentally, to associate the new government with, the Korean economic miracle. Economic growth in Korea was both real and substantial. In 1975, for example, the country's Gross National Product (GNP) in constant (1982) dollars was $44.3 billion. Five years later, in 1980, it was $63.1 billion. During the same period, per capita income, though modest by world standards, rose from $1,207 to $1,586. By 1983, three years into the Chun administration, real GNP reached $77.4

billion and per capita GNP was $1,870. The value of Korean exports, a mere $55 million in 1962, exceeded $26 billion by 1983. By 1980, 57 percent of the country's population resided in urban areas, and by 1985, Seoul, home to nearly one Korean in four, ranked as the ninth most populous urban center in the world. While lagging in development by some measures—in 1984, for example, despite a strong (but clearly export-oriented) automobile manufacturing sector, South Korea had one automobile in domestic use for every eighty-nine of its citizens compared with a 1:4 ratio in Japan and a 1:16 ratio in Mexico)—it was evident in 1980 that the economic tide in the country was on the rise, and that Korea's role in world trade was growing in importance.[2] In this context, the visibility afforded by a successful Olympic enterprise would proclaim to the world South Korea's new status as an industrializing country while providing a vehicle for credit claiming at home.

It followed from this economic success story that increasing numbers of Korean citizens were acquiring an economic stake in political stability. This gave rise to the second impetus to bidding for the Olympics, the opportunity it would provide to associate the government with the intense national pride sure to accompany selection and the preparations for the games. At a time of great political stress, the government clearly hoped that the prospect of losing the games because of political instability once Seoul had been selected as their site would buy for it a window of opportunity to broaden its base of political support. Indeed, as a symbolic statement of the boost to its confidence the Olympic selection afforded, some two months later (December 1981) the government lifted a nationwide curfew that had been in effect since the end of World War II.

Finally, the administration saw a need to confront the perceived threat from North Korea and the issue of reunification. The bonds of race, language, and traditional culture between north and south on the Korean peninsula are strong, but they are matched by the intensity of the animosity between the two states. So volatile and so difficult is the reunification question, in fact, that public discussion of the issue was banned outright by successive governments prior to the administration of President Roh Tae Woo.[3] With some cause, the Chun government viewed the regime of Kim Il Sung in the north as a threat to its continuity and to political stability in the south. With less evident cause, it also viewed North Korea as a threat to the continued success of the South Korean economy. But the government was concerned that the external visibility and credibility of its perceived vulnerability to hostile action from the north was diminishing, as evidenced by the moves to withdraw U.S. military forces from the peninsula during the Carter administration. The government's hope was that, by focusing world attention on South Korea for the better part of a decade, it would reap two benefits. First, the government would have an opportunity to renew world awareness about the North Korean threat. Second, South Korea would purchase a form of insurance against northern aggression. The Olympics were seen as a means to both ends.

Viewed from the perspective of the Korean government in 1980, then, the logic of bidding to host the 1988 Olympic games was apparent. The games would provide legitimacy at home and protection from a hostile sister state, and they would serve notice to the world of Korea's arrival as an economic power.

The "Japanese Model"

In developing these expectations, the Koreans were tantalized by what they thought of as the "Japanese model" of Olympic politics. Korea's relationship with Japan can truly be described as a love–hate one. The Japanese occupied the Korean peninsula for much of this century, earning a good deal of enmity in the process. At the same time, however, Koreans recognize the unparalleled economic growth of postwar Japan and have adapted some Japanese development techniques to their own needs. While distrusting and disliking their neighboring island state, they nevertheless appreciate and emulate much that is Japanese and aspire to rival Japan as an economic power.

In the present instance, the Japanese model in question was that of the Tokyo Olympic Games of 1964, which are generally regarded as the coming out party of the Japanese economy (Espy, 1979: 76). The Korean government's fascination with this model, and its hope to replicate the Japanese experience in Seoul in 1988, led them either to ignore the political risks to the regime entailed in creating an Olympic event or to accept them willingly. The evidence on this question, to which we shall return below, is mixed. In either case, the *designation* of Seoul on October 1, 1981, as host city for the 1988 games itself appears to have been a watershed political event.

The Japanese model is an interesting one in this context and worthy of some elaboration. There is no need here to review in detail the growth of the Japanese economy in the postwar period and its development into a major force in world trade. Suffice it to say that the initial stages of that growth predated the 1964 Olympics, and that in the years since, the Japanese economy has continued to develop and mature. What may be of more interest in the present instance are the concomitant trends in the development of Japan's image as a key player in world affairs.

Figure 6.1 illustrates these trends using two indicators of the volume of news coverage of Japan in the United States for the period 1959 (five

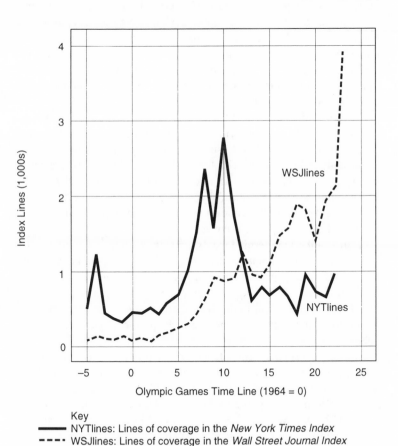

Figure 6.1. Prominence of political and economic news: Japan, 1959–87

years before the Tokyo Olympics) through 1987. The first of these is the total number of lines of references to Japan in the *New York Times Index* year by year. The *Times,* of course, is well established as a principal source of information for the U.S. political elite, so a measure of the weight assigned by the newspaper to news of Japan offers a good esti-mate of the relative *political* importance of Japan on the policymakers' agenda.[4] The second measure summarizes the lines of references to Japan in the *Wall Street Journal Index,* which abstracts a principal source of information for the U.S. economic elite, also aggregated by year. Insofar as *Journal* coverage of foreign affairs is allocated accord-ing to the apparent economic importance of a given country, these data constitute a rough measure of Japan's *economic* significance to the United States through the same period.[5]

From Figure 6.1 four points are clear. First, Japan's apparent political importance during this period was more erratic than its economic impor-tance in that it was more subject to peaks and valleys and less easily characterized by a consistent trend. This should not be surprising since political import is potentially more event determined and less dependent on a secularly developed infrastructure than is economic import.

Second, and consistent with the notion of the Olympics as a rite of passage, though Japanese economic growth had begun much earlier, it was not until shortly after the Tokyo games were staged in 1964 that the long upward trend in economic coverage began, accompanied briefly by a similar takeoff in political coverage.[6]

Third, in the long term, Japan's apparent economic importance has surpassed its political importance, and the gap appears to be widening. This, too, should not be surprising since the Japanese have only a minimal military force and prefer to pursue low visibility strategies in world affairs other than trade. Indeed, it was not until mid-1988 that Japan decided to seek a higher political profile (Hiatt and Shapiro, 1988).

Fourth, in absolute terms, Japan is very prominent in economic re-porting. By the end of the observation period, for example, in the *Wall Street Journal Index* references to Japan filled fifteen pages *per year.*

. A fifth point is suggested by Figure 6.1 but emerges more clearly in Figure 6.2. One way to assess the relationship between two variables such as the levels of political and economic news of Japan is to plot corresponding values against one another on a scatter diagram like that in Figure 6.2—in effect, graphically to ask the question: What level of

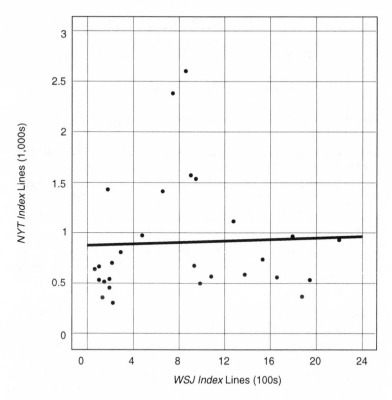

Figure 6.2. Regression of *New York Times Index* lines on *Wall Street Journal Index* lines: Japan, 1959–87

annual coverage of political news do we find for each corresponding level of annual coverage of economic news? Then we look for a straight line that effectively summarizes any pattern that emerges. Such a line is called a regression line, and the degree to which it satisfactorily summarizes the relationship between the two variables—it's ''goodness of fit,'' or the tightness with which the individual points of correspondence on the scatter diagram cluster around the line—is captured in a statistic known as the correlation coefficient.

Figure 6.2 summarizes the regression of political news on economic news for Japan for the 1959–87 time period. Since the observations are widely disbursed around the line, we conclude that the regression line does not provide a good estimate of the data, or, in other words, that the two variables—political and economic news—are independent of one another. Not surprisingly, the correlation coefficient (r) for this association is a very low .05.

The implication of this result is that Japan's apparent political importance has not kept pace with the centrality of its perceived economic role. Put another way, the country has achieved acceptance of its economic legitimacy without substantial world attention being focused on its political system or noneconomic policies. Though it is unlikely that the Chun administration applied this particular methodology to its decision making, it is well to remember that, in image terms, Korea's emerging strength was essentially economic in character, while its continuing vulnerability was political. Thus it may be no coincidence that the Korean Olympic bid came five years after Japan's economic significance emerged as the predominant characteristic of its news image.

While economic independence and approbation were heady objectives in themselves, the political elements of the Japanese model may also have held some allure for the Koreans. The Japan of 1964 was (and in 1980 remained) a one-party, democratic, corporatist East Asian state not entirely unlike that which President Chun may have intended to bequeath to his successor. The same party had controlled Japanese politics since pre-Olympic days and had received much of the political credit for the economic advances of that period. Moreover, the news of Japan in 1964 was on balance quite favorable. The country's economic growth rate was projected at twice that of other advanced countries, taxes were cut (though inflation was a problem), and the first cautious steps were taken toward normalizing relations with the Peoples Republic of China. The Olympics were portrayed by the government as a source of economic benefit for the country and as a symbolic welcoming back of Japan into the family of nations. There was a split within the ruling party over increasing Japan's international role, but calls for a policy of "economic diplomacy," a renewed world role, and a better sense of direction in regional affairs predominated. Above all, there was little external news of political dissent, and the only political violence was an apparently nonpolitical stabbing of U.S. Ambassador Edwin Reischauer. The games themselves were conducted without incident and succeeded in drawing much positive attention to the host country.

For all of its attractiveness, however, there were situational differences that might have called into question the applicability of the Japanese model of the 1960s to Korea in the 1980s. The continued pressure generated by the presence of an aggressive and hostile regime north of the Demilitarized Zone (DMZ), the generally greater distrust of governmental authority extant among the Korean people, the residual bitterness born of the violence at Kwangju and the repression of opposition leaders, the confrontational character of Korean political dialogue—these and other factors held the potential to render the Japanese model inoperative. Indeed, events of 1987 and 1988, products of these forces, pointed toward an altogether different and far less flattering model, that provided by the Mexico City Olympics of 1968.

The "Mexican Model"

Though Americans probably best remember the 1968 games for the clenched-fist black power salute of medalists Tommie Smith and John Carlos during the playing of the *Star Spangled Banner,* the most compelling political aspect of the Mexico City Olympics was the two years of political instability and street violence that preceded the games. Table 6.1 presents a chronology of these events.

Table 6.1. Chronology of Political Instability in Mexico: 1967–68

Date	Event
1967	
March 23	11 killed and at least 35 injured in three days of rioting by students in Hermosillo protesting a ruling PRI gubernatorial nomination. (Mexican police are supplied with tear gas by the state of Arizona, whose governor describes the act as part of his "good neighbor policy.")
May	Students in Sonora state strike and close university.
May 20	Parents of striking students rally in support of the strike.
July 3	PRI sweeps elections, winning 87 percent of vote, all 178 contested deputy's seats, all 7 gubernatorial races.
July 11	Opposition party, PAN, charges PRI with voting irregularities.
July 19–20	Government arrests 13 in plot allegedly backed by Peoples Republic of China through its Hsinhua news agency office to overthrow the Mexican government; discloses conspiracy to train rural and urban terrorists at jungle camps; seizes 12 tons of propaganda materials; searches schools for students who reportedly pledged to join guerilla movement.

(continued)

Table 6.1. Chronology of Political Instability in Mexico: 1967–68
(*continued*)

Date	Event
1967	
September 21	A split in a key union in the PRI coalition leads to violence in Acapulco with 21 killed.
1968	
July 26	2,000 students rampage through Mexico City demanding ouster of mayor and chief of riot police: 1 killed, 400 injured.
July 30	Students riot in Mexico City to protest brutality of police in previous riot; dispersed by riot police; government blames Communist youth organization; journalists assaulted by police; U.S. embassy defaced by antigovernment slogans.
July 31	Student demonstrations spread to two state capitals; troops move in; 2 reported killed in riot in Villahermosa; government charges that many of those arrested are foreign agitators.
August 1	50,000 demonstrators march peacefully in Mexico City to protest police brutality and violation of university autonomy.
August 3	President Diaz calls for conciliation, joint commission of inquiry.
August 9	15,000 students start general strike; student organizations reject government call for inquiry.
August 10	Thousands of students march through Mexico City, stage sit-in in front of National Palace; object to being labeled "Communists."
August 21	Students and young professionals protest economic, social, political, and cultural conditions; call for formation of new party and major street demonstration.
August 27	200,000 students, teachers and parents march on president's office; demand freeing of political prisoners; movement fails to attract broader support.
August 28	Riot police with bayonets clear 3,000 students from Constitution Square area
September 13	Students march in Mexico City; refuse request to halt demonstrations during Olympic Games.
September 19	Army seizes control of National University in Mexico City; students and police clash in several areas of city.
September 21	Government frees 250 students arrested earlier, forms commission to review grievances; several thousand students clash with police in Mexico City.

Table 6.1. (*continued*)

Date	Event
1968	
September 22	Major street fighting in Mexico City as students seize National Polytechnic Institute.
September 23	Street fighting continues as police storm campus; thousands of students march on prison to free fellow students.
September 23–24	Battle rages over Polytechnic Institute campus; first use of firearms by students; students lose building but stage large rally nearby; government begins prosecuting rioters; student actions win sympathy but no support from major PRI constituencies.
September 24	Government assures International Olympic Committee situation will be under control by October 12 start of games.
September 25	Center of Mexico City under state of siege.
September 27	Students rally near Polytechnic Institute.
September 29	Government agrees to restructure commission of inquiry; both sides express desire to avoid incidents during Olympics.
September 30	Troops withdraw from National University, but remain at Polytechnic Institute and other schools; mothers of slain students march through city.
October 1	Students vow to continue strike; plan no demonstrations during Olympics.
October 2	Troops fire on rally of 3,000; at least 49 killed including 6 members of the students' national strike committee.
October 3	Students burn three trolley buses; Olympic officials announce intention to start games on schedule.
October 5	Demonstrations held in Monterrey and Aguascalientes.
October 9	Government and students discuss ending conflict; students reject talks.
October 12	Olympic Games open under heavy security.
October 29	Student injured in clash with soldiers; government releases more than 100 students from prison.
November 8	Students vote to continue strike.
November 22	Student leaders call for return to classes.
November 27	Students battle over return to classes; 1 killed, 30 injured.
December 4	National Student Council declares end to strike.
December 24	Government releases 121 students; moves to lower voting age, simplify release of political detainees; aims for reconciliation with students.

Source: *New York Times Index*, 1967, 1968.

The similarity between this chronology and the sequence of events in South Korea beginning in the spring of 1987 is, at least at first blush, quite striking. In Korea, as in Mexico, students engaged in long-running confrontations with riot police and staged large-scale demonstrations in the heart of the national capital to press their demands for reform. Police responded with shows of force; students and police were injured; campuses were closed by student strikes and government action; charges of outside agitation (this time by North Korea) were leveled. Beyond the apparent parallelism of events, there were as well some superficial structural similarities. In both instances, the initiative, organization and ''staffing'' of the demonstrations was left to university students. Both countries had been dominated by a single political party; both had had weak and fractured oppositions. In addition, both countries had been economically dependent on the United States.

But there are significant differences between these two cases as well.

- Though the scale of demonstrations in Korea was much larger, for example, than that in Mexico, the level of violence associated with them was much lower, at least to the extent that far fewer persons were killed. Indeed, Korean riot police did not use firearms in quelling disturbances, while Mexican authorities used them rather freely.
- Though the student movement in Mexico failed ultimately to ignite participatory support among other constituencies, notably labor, that in South Korea did succeed to some extent in broadening its base. Some members of the Korean middle class gave signs of support, and during the summer of 1987, Korean labor took to the streets to call for enhanced workers' rights.
- Though both countries have been single-party dominated, the PRI in Mexico claims a revolutionary heritage, and its principal *electoral* competition is from the right. The ruling Democratic Justice Party (DJP) (since renamed following a merger with two opposition parties) in Korea had a military heritage and faced its principal electoral competition from the left. This difference may account for the ability of protesting Korean students to generate support from opposition politicians, which Mexican protestors were unable to do.
- In addition, though both countries have been economically depen-

dent on the United States, their economies, and the nature of their dependency, differ. The Korean economy of 1987–88 was far stronger and growing more rapidly than that of Mexico in 1968, and it relied on the United States to absorb its exports of manufactured goods. Mexico's principal export to the United States, on the other hand, was its labor force, and the major emphasis of the late 1960s was on the establishment of *maquiladoras,* U.S.-owned factories in border communities that would be granted special export concessions in an effort to generate an industrial base in northern Mexico.

- Finally, unlike the demonstrators in Mexico in 1968, those in Korea in 1987 won significant concessions from the government. The electoral system was changed; the Constitution was redrawn; and in legislative elections in early 1988, the DJP lost its control of a newly strengthened National Assembly.

One other aspect of the Mexico model is worthy of note before we conclude this portion of our discussion, a comparison of the post-Olympic news image of Mexico with that of Japan. Using methodology similar to that for the analysis of news space devoted to Japan in the *New York Times* and the *Wall Street Journal,* Figures 6.3 and 6.4 illustrate the importance attached to Mexico by American journalists during the period 1963 to 1987. Figure 6.3 shows the aggregated levels of coverage in each newspaper, while Figure 6.4 represents the regression of *Times* coverage on that in the *Journal.* As before, year zero in Figure 6.3 represents the Olympic year, in this case 1968.

What is striking here in comparison with the Japanese case is the close and continuing relationship between political and economic coverage. This is apparent from a visual inspection of Figure 6.3, which shows that the levels of political and economic coverage track closely with one another over the years, and from a glance at the distribution of observations around the regression line in Figure 6.4, which shows considerable clustering. Indeed, the correlation coefficient (r) here is .69, indicating that economic news may account for as much as 47 percent of the variance in political coverage.[7] A more complete, multivariate analysis would probably show this figure to be inflated, but there can be no doubt that a fundamental difference does exist in the magnitude of this association from the Mexican to the Japanese model.

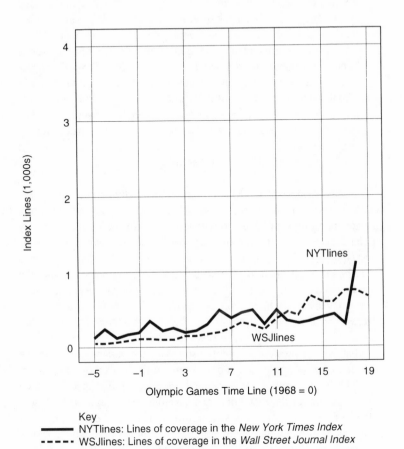

Figure 6.3. Prominence of political and economic news: Mexico, 1963–87

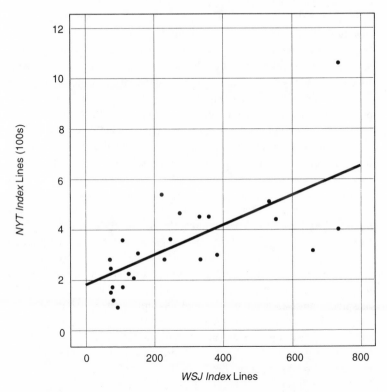

Figure 6.4. Regression of *New York Times Index* lines on *Wall Street Journal Index* lines: Mexico, 1963–87

Seoul 1988: Japan, Mexico, or Korea?

Which, in the end, was the operative model most applicable to the Seoul Olympics? Which helps us best to understand the events of the period and project their consequences? Let us consider two key elements of these questions, the economic and the political, in turn.

Economically, South Korea in the 1980s resembled much more closely the Japan of 1964 than it did the Mexico of 1968. It had a well-established industrial sector, a vigorous work force, and a strong foothold in world markets for durable goods. It was developing a well-educated and large middle class, and the standard of living of its people had risen steadily. The Korean currency, the *won,* was aggressively prevented from rising against the U.S. dollar to protect the country's share of U.S. markets for textiles, automobiles, and other goods, and, as in Japan, import barriers had been erected to protect domestic industries. Indeed, Korea's economic importance as reflected in its *Wall Street Journal* coverage was already more than double that afforded to Japan at a comparable point on the Olympics time line. And, despite labor unrest over the two years preceeding the Olympics, the work force remained not only highly productive, but tractable. In June 1988, for example, a two-month strike against Hyundai auto plants was called off by union leaders for the stated reason that it was hurting the company.

On the political front, South Korea bore a superficial resemblance to the Mexican model, especially with respect to the temporal development of student protests leading up to the Olympic Games. As in Mexico, there had been numerous violent clashes, and there was evident a residue of bitter distrust of the government among university students. But there the similarity ended. For in Korea the protest and pressure for democratization could be seen as the products of a crisis of rising expectations, a lag between the political needs of an increasingly affluent population and the willingness of their governing elite to open the political process to broader participation. In Mexico, the violence that erupted in 1968 was, if anything, the product of a crisis of no expectations, of a moribund governmental bureaucracy unable to respond to fundamental economic and social problems.

Indeed, what may be most interesting about the denouement in South Korea is the role played by the Olympics as a catalyst for political change. If it was the government's intention in part to use the games to enhance its own legitimacy, that strategy may well have backfired. In any event, it is clear in retrospect that, in the summer of 1987, the Korean government found itself between the proverbial rock—student demonstrators—and a hard place of its own making—the 1988 Seoul Olympics. It may or may not have been the anticipation of the Olympics that brought students into the streets in June 1987, but it was surely the anticipation of the Olympics that brought the world's press to Seoul, Kwangju, and elsewhere to cover their activities. And it was the presence of the press, the negative image of South Korea it conveyed to the world, and the legitimacy it conferred on demonstrators and opposition politicians that ultimately forced the ruling party to make significant political concessions. The Olympics were a symbol bestowed with great importance by the government—through huge countdown clocks posted around Seoul, banners and ceremonies, traffic control practice sessions, and numerous promotional campaigns—but they were a symbol over which the government lost control. Rather than a pressure point for sustaining the political status quo to maintain stability, they became a pressure point forcing controlled change to maintain stability. In effect, the Olympic countdown marked a deadline for a restructuring of the political system.

One effect that the hosting of the Olympics probably did have that was among the Chun government's initial objectives was the affording of some protection from, and the further isolation of, North Korea. The hard bargaining over a northern role as a venue for several Olympic events, the unwavering support of the IOC for South Korea's status as sole host, and the public outcry after North Korean agents bombed a Korean Air flight, strengthened the south's hand in dealing with its neighbor. It may, in fact, be the case that the benefits gained from hosting the 1988 games contributed materially to the subsequent progress toward reunification with the north that has long been a central objective of all Korean governments.

Implications for Political
Communication Research

While the characterization of the role of the Seoul Olympics in the political and economic development of the host country may be an interesting exercise in its own right, it is of lasting import primarily insofar as it yields larger insights into the uses of the Olympics and other, similar bundles of prominent condensation symbols—those around which a government, leader, or political movement can stir emotions and mobilize support or opposition—in international and domestic political communication. In this regard, the Korean experience suggests several tentative conclusions around which discussion might focus. Among them:

- The Olympic Games and other similarly magnetic events do have the potential to play a cathartic role in the political lives of nations. In this assumption, the Chun administration appears to have been correct. As a prism through which the outside world viewed the Republic of Korea, and as a focal point for domestic political attention, the Seoul Olympics proved an effective generator of visibility and political awareness.

- The Olympic Games are, in fact, so potent as a political symbol that the host government has been unable to maintain control over their impact. As was the case in Mexico two decades earlier, the substantial investment of governmental prestige in the success of the Olympics created in South Korea an artificial but overwhelming pressure on the government itself to sustain the national pride that is so much a part of hosting the games. The advent of the games effectively forced the government to confront basic questions of political development, which were not initially on its own near-term agenda and whose resolution appears to have been contrary to the defined interests of the ruling party.

- As the events of 1987 to 1988 in South Korea unfolded, the unusual outside attention brought to bear on them because of the impending Olympics added to the pressures on the Korean government to formulate a response sufficient to defuse its opposition and probably increased the likelihood that the response, when it came, represented a movement toward further democratization. Visits by IOC representatives and indications that some athletes were considering absenting themselves from the games surely added to the pressure from the United States and other governments to undertake fundamental political reform.

- In all of this, the international news media played the role of catalyst in both the domestic and international exchanges that led to political change in South Korea in advance of the Olympic Games. Though I have argued elsewhere (Manheim, 1988a, 1988b) that

Western media could have done a more effective job of developing their audience's understanding of events in Korea during the summer of 1987, there can be little doubt that the images they did create played a central role in framing the Korean question for external audiences and in pressing reform on the government. Moreover, the knowledge that their actions were attracting world attention, which was translating into pressure on their government, gave added impetus to student demonstrators and opposition politicians alike.

We will see evidence in Chapter 7 that efforts by governments to improve their portrayal in the news media of other states can succeed when low visibility strategies are pursued, but are far less likely to result in favorable image shifts when dramatic historical events, political violence, or overt evidence of the image-enhancement efforts themselves intervene. In this context, it might be useful to view the hosting of the Olympics as a highly dramatic, highly visible, quasi-historical, intermediate-length event that possesses a sufficient dynamic of its own, under certain circumstances, to overwhelm those who would use or control it. As such, the act of hosting the Olympics—or of staging any similar mega-event—entails not only a set of potentially attractive opportunities for any government contemplating it, but a set of readily predictable and appreciable political risks as well.

III

Analysis and Implications

7

Managing National Images

In the previous section, we examined several instances in which governments sought, with greater or lesser strategic sophistication and with greater or lesser effectiveness, to manage the images of them extant among the media, the public, and the foreign policy elites of other nations, most notably the United States. We considered the formal diplomatic practices that provide a framework for some of these efforts and the inherent tendency of the media to paint regionally stereotyped pictures for their audiences. And we reviewed some of the efforts of countries like Kuwait, Pakistan, and South Korea to enhance their images abroad in the hope of gaining some economic or political advantage. In this section, and especially in the present chapter, we will turn our attention to a more formal and essentially quantitative analysis of some aspects of such efforts at image management. In the process, we will also move from the tactical level to the strategic, focusing less on the particular activities undertaken in a given instance and more on the underlying rationale that gives direction to the selection and bundling of such activities in one circumstance or another.

One word of caution is in order. The nature of the argument to this point has readily lent itself to a descriptive style of narrative that, I hope, no reader has found unduly imposing. In Chapters 7 and 8, however, the analysis takes a rather different form, and the challenge of conveying it in the requisite detail without loss of clarity becomes much greater. I promise to give this a good effort, but I also ask the reader's indulgence if the presentation becomes, to some eyes, unduly technical. So that you may have a sense of the terrain that lies ahead, I offer this brief preview of coming attractions:

- The present chapter will set forth a theoretical perspective that both explains and predicts the strategies that will be selected by image-management consultants serving foreign governments, with the selection itself to be determined by the characteristics of the client's image at the beginning of the effort. The theory is tested by predicting the changes in news portrayals of several countries as a result of their initiating image-management efforts, then comparing these predictions against actual measures of media content.
- Chapter 8 builds on this analysis by presenting a more general model of the relationships among media, the public, and policymakers—termed the "Model of Agenda Dynamics"—and suggests the ways this model can be used to improve our understanding of information flows in the political and policy arenas.
- Chapter 9, which features a return to the less technical narrative style of the previous sections, identifies and discusses issues related both to the scholarly questions raised by the arguments and analysis of this book and to the very challenging political questions associated with the practice of U.S.-directed strategic political communication in the international arena.

Academic readers will want to press ahead through the full development of the argument. Others may prefer to sample the wares in the present chapter, then move to Chapter 9.

Controlling the Foreign Policy Agenda

Each participant in the process of making or implementing public policy—or in the present instance, foreign policy—is seen by students of such activity to have what is termed an "agenda"—a set of concerns or preferences that are drawing attention at a particular point in time. These agendas are seen, essentially, as more or less open systems loosely connected with one another, so that concerns or preferences can move from one to the next—from the media's agenda to the public's, from the public's agenda to that of the policymakers, and so forth. This exchange of content is described in the literature variously as ''agenda setting'' or ''agenda building'' and has attracted a great deal of scholarly attention.

A common assumption in much of the social science research on setting or building agendas is that, whatever the nature of the exchanges among the media, the public, and political elites, the external context in which interaction occurs is neutral, or at the very least, benign. On this or that issue, public opinion may be more or less susceptible to menu writing by the media, or policymakers may be more or less responsive to mediated messages or constituency contacts. But no outside parties are considered to be at work to alter the process of exchange itself—to manipulate the behavior of the media, the public, or the political leadership as they pass agenda items back and forth among themselves.

But as any lobbyist or political consultant will tell us, and any political scientist should know by instinct, the process is hardly so pristine. In reality, many people make a good living disrupting stasis in the system of agendas.

That is no less true in foreign affairs than in domestic politics or policymaking. As Page and Shapiro (1983), Graber (1988), and others have demonstrated, the internal forces of agenda setting function in foreign affairs much as they do in other areas. In fact, the manipulation of news and public images of actors and events in foreign affairs is actually more likely to have an effect than it is in the domestic sphere. This is the case for at least three reasons.

First, the issues and actors in foreign affairs are, in Eyal's (1980) term, unobtrusive. That is to say, the public is relatively unlikely to have any direct experience related to issues in foreign policy of the sort they might very well have on the domestic side. Many Americans will feel the results of an economic slowdown accompanied by a wave of job layoffs, but few will personally experience the results of an increase in economic assistance to Russia of a billion dollars or the sale to Pakistan of a dozen jet fighters. As a result, any widely held public opinion that develops on issues of foreign policy is likely to be heavily media dependent—media being the only available source of information about the issue—and, as a consequence, simplified and relatively homogeneous.

Second, the media themselves are limited in both their ability and their inclination to devote staff and resources to covering news of foreign affairs. Their ability is limited because of the proportionately greater expense, and the sheer logistical difficulty, of providing substantial coverage of foreign affairs except from domestic venues such as the Department of State or the United Nations. Their inclination is limited because audience interest in foreign affairs is so low that news organizations have no incentive to invest the additional resources that would be required to enhance their coverage. In comparison with domestic coverage, this produces news that is limited to a few sources providing information on a few stories that are conveyed through a few centralized channels (Becker, 1977).

Third, even public officials can have a difficult time gathering information about many aspects of foreign affairs, so even they may be dependent on the media in some measure—if not for event-specific information, at the least for general impressions of various countries or regions (Cohen, 1973; Sigal, 1973). And in today's environment of instantaneous electronic dissemination of news, as we have already noted, the media clearly limit the opportunities available to decision makers for patience and careful reflection.

Together, these observations add up to an opportunity for influence, a collection of vulnerabilities to outside intervention that are inherent in many foreign affairs related issues and events. Combined with a motive that is apparent from the scale and influence of the U.S. role in world affairs, they offer a rough contour map of the ground on which U.S.-directed strategic public diplomacy is practiced.

In the present context, the media agenda is worthy of special attention because its decisions, more than those of the public or the policymakers, relate directly to information flows and because its principal political role is to serve as a conduit between the other two sets of participants. It is also an agenda to which those who would influence foreign policy attend closely. From studies of cross-national newspaper advertising by national governments (Amaize and Faber, 1983) as well as direct examination of the Foreign Agent Registration Act (FARA) filings with the Department of Justice, we know that substantial resources are devoted to shaping these media portrayals.

Figure 7.1 summarizes these efforts at intervention in the foreign affairs agenda system. The three boxes representing the media, public, and policy agendas actually stand for some rather complex processes that we will examine more closely in Chapter 8. For the moment, let us think of them simply as the list of policy concerns that are drawing the attention of each group, respectively, at a given time. The fourth box, labeled ''External Influences,'' represents the efforts of public diplo-

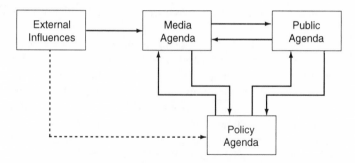

Figure 7.1. Public relations and agenda setting

matists to influence the system by either of two means. The broken line running to the policy agenda represents efforts at direct lobbying by American firms in behalf of foreign clients, or direct contacts by representives of foreign governments with their U.S. counterparts. As indicated earlier, such lobbying is not the primary focus of the present analysis, though it certainly accompanies many of the efforts at image management that constitute our primary concern. The solid line running to the media agenda represents efforts at indirect influence, that which is channeled to the policymakers through the media and, in some instances, secondarily through their constituents. It is the effect on media portrayals of these attempts at influence that will provide the focus for the balance of the present chapter.

Media Coverage and Media Management

In general, long-term patterns of foreign news coverage in the United States have been found to vary in association with such factors as the levels of trade and telecommunications traffic between the United States and the nation in question, that nation's overall status or importance in the world, the population of the country, the apparent national interest of the United States, the occurence of crises, and the problems posed by foreign censors (Charles, Shore, and Todd, 1979; Lent, 1977; Peterson, 1981). We saw some evidence of these patterns in the analysis of regional variations in dominant news frames presented in Chapter 5. With the possible exception of crises, these factors establish a baseline of news coverage of a given country around which variations occur.

It is not my objective here to explain this baseline coverage. Rather, the present analysis takes this baseline of differential media interest in various countries as a given and focuses on variations around the baseline that have two elements in common. First, they are systematic in the sense that each variation represents what might reasonably be believed to be nonrandom fluctuations. Second, they are associated in time with a specific class of event, the introduction of a news- or image-management campaign by a U.S. consultant working in behalf of a foreign government.

As one might expect, these "public relations" interventions can include such services as the preparation and distribution of press kits, direct mailings, newsletters, video press releases, brochures—in short, the full range of informational flotsam and jetsam commonly associated in the public mind with image doctoring. But such services are not among the most significant provided by image consultants, and they may even be used at times as distractions. Much more important are the efforts at news management and control over the flow of client-related information. Consultants routinely train embassy personnel in the workings and news values of American news organizations and counsel them on how to discuss such problems as terrorism or human rights violations or economic instability. They schedule or conduct field trips for the press to areas of the client country to which they wish to call attention and help to restrict access to those they wish avoided. They organize the visits of foreign dignitaries and assure that they meet Americans of interest, and they provide or restrict access of U.S. and other journalists to key officials of the client government. Using their own networks of contacts—many are former journalists or government officials—they help representatives of the client states develop personal relationships with U.S. journalists or government officials. And, drawing on both their own expertise and a full range of research services, they help their clients to package their own policies in ways that will make them palatable to relevant U.S. constituencies. The question at hand is whether any of this makes a difference, at least with respect to media portrayals.

To answer that question, during the 1980s Robert Albritton and I developed a series of studies employing a technique known as interrupted time series analysis applied to content analytic data on media coverage of foreign countries. Interrupted time series analysis can be used whenever a long-running series of observations is impacted by an experimental event or intervention of some sort. It permits us to estimate the effect that this intervention has on the behavior we have been observing.

In the present instance, the dependent variables—the behaviors we were observing over the long term—were image attributes of the news portrayals of several countries that we knew had hired American image consultants. The independent variable in each instance—the outside event whose impact on news portrayals we were attempting to measure—was the FARA-registered initiation of the public relations contract for each client country, which we treated as an intervention in the time series. In essence, we compared levels and trends in the news coverage of each country between the year immediately preceeding the signing of the contract and the year immediately following. In the balance of this chapter, I will describe this research in a bit more detail and will summarize our findings. For a complete analysis, the reader is referred to the original reports of this research, which are listed in the bibliography.

Modeling Communication Strategies

Drawing on the logic that later came to underlie development of the full agenda-dynamics model presented in the next chapter, we determined that two aspects of the media image of foreign countries were of special importance in framing the perceptions and actions of U.S. policymakers who might be successfully influenced. The first, visibility, refers to the amount of media coverage that a given country receives. The second, valence, refers to the degree to which the content that is available reflects either favorably or unfavorably on the country in question. The relationship between these two dimensions of news portrayals is summarized in Figure 7.2.

In the figure, visibility is represented by location along the vertical axis and valence by location along the horizontal axis. This produces four quadrants, each of which represents a more or less unique setting that defines the objectives of the intervention. In the northwest quadrant, for example, are found countries that are frequently the subject of news coverage, but whose images are generally negative. News coverage of Iraq during the Persian Gulf Crisis or South Africa over the past two

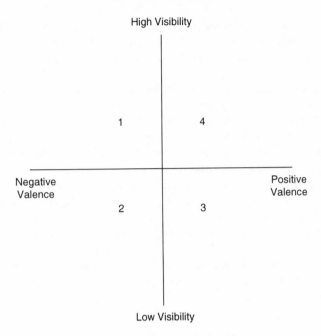

Figure 7.2. Dimensions of national image

decades would be examples of such highly visible, negatively valenced coverage. Portrayals of this type are likely to be accompanied by relatively high degrees of public awareness of the client country and of its projected image (Benton and Frazier, 1976). Under these conditions, explicit efforts to portray a country in a positive light are likely to be rejected, by the media and public alike, as propaganda in the most pejorative sense (Merritt, 1980; Wolfsfeld, 1983). Productive image management in this region of the figure, then, will necessarily be restricted principally to affecting positioning on the visibility dimension, where the objective would be to bring about a reduction that may facilitate later efforts directed at improving the valence component of the country's image.

In the southwest quadrant, circumstances are rather different. Here we have countries whose portrayals may be at least as negative, on balance, as those in the northwest, but where media (and public) attention is considerably less. Historically, we might find here such countries as Pakistan or the Philippines. Especially as we approach the lowest levels of visibility, we encounter conditions very much like those that Krugman (1965) has described as conducive to low-involvement learning, that in which an audience is influenced not by persuasion and reason, but by the circumventing of its normal psychological defenses against new, discrepant information, and that Wolfsfeld (1983) has characterized as the most conducive to effective persuasion through international propaganda.

Whether it is the journalists themselves (and, therefore, the content of the media agenda) who are rendered more susceptible, or whether, through the operation of classic agenda setting, it is the public that is so rendered, the opportunities for reconfiguring the valence of a client country's news image are substantial in this quadrant. Eyal (1980) has suggested that most issues and actors in foreign policy would, in fact, display low levels of news visibility and of public awareness, and many of the countries whose images we have examined in the years since he wrote have resided in these depths of not only relative, but absolute, invisibility.

Passing across Figure 7.2 from west to east, one crosses the boundary between what Bernard Cohen (1973) once termed reactive manipulation and active manipulation. Rather than constantly putting out fires, the consultant has opportunities here to develop a positive image for the client. Switzerland would be typical of countries found in the southeast quadrant, while Great Britain would generally fall in the northeast. Both countries, of course, have potential negatives—Switzerland with its highly restrictive political system, and Great Britain with its depressed economy and associated racial and social unrest. But in each instance, attention to problems is generally outweighed by more positive portrayals, and it is the image, not the reality, that is at issue here.

Because countries in these quadrants start from a more favored position, the focus of their public relations activity is more likely to be on increasing visibility and further enhancing valence so as to reinforce their existing, and desirable, images. It is here that overt promotional efforts can make a positive contribution to image enhancement. But even here, these may be tactical rather than strategic tools and are scarcely among the most advanced techniques available. A more sophisticated approach might be one derived, for example, from McGuire's (1964) notion of inoculation against attitude change.[1] In such a strategy, members of the audience—which in this instance might be actors on any

of the three agendas—are immunized against negative slippage in their
image of the client country through such persuasive themes and devices
as the forging of links between the image in question and some valued
goal of the public or the individual in question,[2] or by encouraging
public expressions of acceptance of the image. The latter, for example,
is a strategy employed regularly by Israel, which elicits statements of
support from policymakers and other persons, the issuance of which
increases both the political and the psychological cost of reducing support from the stated levels. Recall that the U.S. Army employed a
variant of the inoculation strategy to shore up the nation's psychological
defenses against chemical warfare in advance of the 1991 invasion of
Kuwait.

Taken together, these observations suggest a context-sensitive sequence of strategic objectives for would-be image managers. This sequence is represented by the path indicated in Figure 7.3. In the northwest quadrant, where visibility is high and valence is unchangeable, the

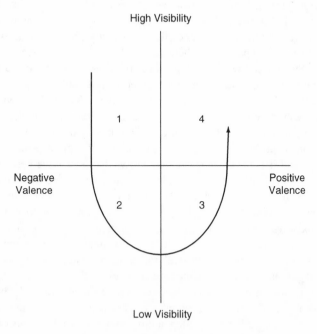

Figure 7.3. Dimensions of national image

objective is to reduce visibility. In the southwest quadrant, where visibility is low and where, as a result, valence is less firmly established, the goal is to improve valence. In the southeast quadrant, where the client's image is good but there is not enough of it, the idea is to increase visibility. And in the northeast quadrant, where both visibility and valence are at desired levels, work to lock them in. The question at hand is whether actual public relations efforts produce effects that are consistent with this pattern.

Testing the Model

To answer that question, we examined news coverage of various countries in the *New York Times* using the general design and approach that I described earlier. We selected the *Times* because it is the most widely read newspaper among elites both within and outside of government (Weiss, 1974) and among the most widely cited by policymakers (Grau, 1976), it has been shown to have a strong agenda-setting effect on public opinion (Winter and Eyal, 1981), it carries a higher volume of foreign news than any other U.S. newspaper (Semmel, 1976), it has been identified specifically as a prefered medium for national-image advertising by foreign governments (Amaize and Faber, 1983), and it is often used as a source of events data by researchers (Hopple, 1982). In addition, precisely because it is atypical of the U.S. press in that it devotes more of its own space and resources to foreign news coverage and is therefore among the most independent of U.S. newspapers in its information gathering, the *New York Times* represents at once a primary target for public relations efforts and an acid test of their effectiveness.

In the initial stages of the research, we identified roughly two dozen countries that had engaged the services of American consultants during the 1970s and early 1980s. We then eliminated from consideration those (indeed, most of the cases) that had such low levels of news coverage that it was not possible to develop meaningful measures of variation on the dependent variables, and those (principally in the Middle East) where events and coverage were so complex that we would be unable to isolate the effects of particular interest. We then focused our analysis on the countries that remained.

For purposes of measurement, visibility was operationalized as the average number of newspaper insertions per month pertaining to a given country. Since, at least in principal, the amount of potential news coverage of a country is open-ended, we arbitrarily set the breakpoint between high and low visibility at thirty per month, or the equivalent of one insertion per day. Thus, by definition, high visibility countries are those that receive, on average, more than one insertion in the *New York Times* per day, and low visibility countries are those that receive fractional coverage. This specification, though arbitrary, appears to have stood us in good stead. And it is the case, in any event, that the strategy suggested in Figure 7.3 is continuous rather than discrete, and interpretation of the results is not solely dependent on placement in specific quadrants.

Valence was defined for our analysis as the percentage of all insertions in a given month that could be characterized as positive or negative with respect to the portrayal of the client country. Positive references included any mention of a country's progress, advances, resources, assets, strengths, continuity, stability, reliability (from a U.S. perspective), or dependability. Negative references included any mention of decline, weakness, poverty, liabilities, lack of progress, instability, or unreliability (from a U.S. perspective) on the part of the country in question.[3] Intercoder reliabilities for measures of visibility and valence, reported in detail in the original documentation, were at acceptable levels.

Our first objective was to test the utility of the basic formulation of the model specified in Figure 7.3. For that purpose, we selected six experimental countries—Argentina, Indonesia, the Republic of Korea, the Philippines, Southern Rhodesia, and Yugoslavia (Turkey was added later)—and one control, Mexico. Mexico was included in the analysis because we were able to document a specific point in time when the Mexican government was approached by an American public relations firm and declined to sign a contract.[4]

The logic of experimentation requires that cases for analysis be drawn in such a manner as to represent some larger population, and that the experimental arrangements be so designed as to rule out alternative explanations for the observed effects. The scale of our research precluded the drawing of a representative sample of countries and time points of public relations intervention, even if this had been possible, and the considerations mentioned above required that cases be eliminated that could not fulfill our measurement requirements. Thus we ended up with what is clearly a judgmental sample.

In addition, when dealing with such small numbers of cases and cases of such idiosyncracy, one must be especially sensitive to unique aspects of each case that might render it meaningless for analysis. Thus, prefatory to conducting the content analysis of news coverage of each experimental country, we reviewed events in each to satisfy ourselves that no event or other unusual circumstance either bound the cases one to another (the resultant interdependence of observations rendering our results meaningless) or provided a plausible rival explanation for the effects we might observe. In our view, all of the cases in the analysis satisfied these criteria.

The results of our initial analysis are summarized in Figure 7.4. For each country whose image is summarized in the figure, the starting point of the visibility/valence vector is defined by the average monthly score on each variable during the year preceeding the contract date (the preintervention period) and the end point by the corresponding averages for the year following the contract date (the postintervention period). Although not all movement in the images of the experimental countries reflected in the figure is in the directions predicted in Figure 7.3, most actually is, and none of that which is contrary in direction achieved statistical significance. There is, in other words, much in Figure 7.4 that confirms our expectations and nothing that significantly disconfirms them. The contradirectional movement in the image of Mexico, our control, adds weight to this conclusion.

At the time we published these results, Albritton and I realized that we might be recording nothing more than multiple cases of a phenomenon known as regression toward the mean, which refers to the natural tendency of statistical series that are testing their extremes to return over time to more central values. It might be argued, for example, that the reason any of these countries sought assistance in the first place was because its image was out of its normal alignment. If all, or most, of the image changes we observed were of this type—if they merely represented movement back toward the "normal" levels of coverage—then the effects we would credit to public relations interventions would be grossly overstated. The strategy we implemented for testing this possibility and eliminating it from consideration is presented in Appendix B.

One of the more intriguing findings in our initial inquiry, and one that added to our confidence that the changes we were observing were neither random nor spurious, was the presence of a time lag of some two to three months between the introduction of the public relations effort and the first shifts in postintervention observational values. Our interpretation is that this time lag, which is consistent across the baseline cases, represents the start-up time for each new image-management effort.

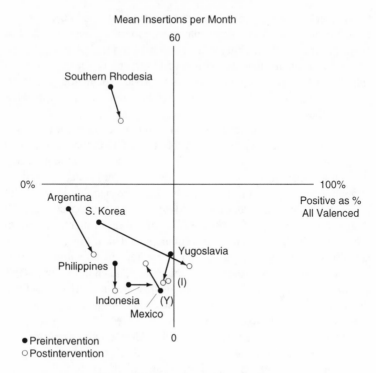

Figure 7.4. Directions of image change

Testing the Limits of the Model

Having established to our satisfaction both the validity of our method and the significance of our findings, we set out to test the limits of our conceptualization of public relations effects. Surely, we felt, such effects would not be demonstrated equally in all circumstances. And we were correct.

Through our research, we determined that at least three factors could limit the potential impact on media or public opinion of an image-management campaign. These include the general visibility of the campaign itself; its association with any sort of controversy; and the presence of contrapuntal, systemic, historical forces. Let us examine an example of each.

Covert Versus Overt Persuasion: The Philippines

Given the grounding of our specification of public relations strategy in the theories of attitude structure and change, it should come as no surprise that the visibility of a persuasive effort per se would minimize its likelihood of success. Public relations consultants are inherently low-credibility sources, and information they may overtly and directly convey to an audience is easily rejected as unduly trustworthy to merit any responding change in attitude. Such efforts may even prove counter-productive, with the audience devaluing its image of the client country precisely because it would engage in such transparent attempts at influence. We find an example of this rejection in a campaign waged by the Philippines circa 1982.

Figure 7.5 summarizes change in news portrayals associated with two efforts undertaken to improve the image in the United States of the Philippines. Like others in this chapter, the figure is based on an analysis of coverage in the *New York Times*. In both instances, the initial image of the Philippines was in the southwest quadrant, that is, low in visibility and generally negative in valence. In the first of these efforts (1977 to 1979, with an intervention in 1978), the government pursued a strategy of image management that produced a statistically significant reduction in visibility, though no improvement in valence. The number and percentage of negative insertions was reduced substantially in the posttest period. But in 1982, in association with an anticipated visit to the United States by then-President Ferdinand Marcos, the Philippine government went to rather extraordinary lengths to doctor its image through an especially *high*-visibility campaign. The result was rather different.

The effort was begun in the spring of 1982. In preparation for his visit, Marcos assigned a new ambassador to the Philippine embassy in Washington, Benjamin Romualdez—his wife's brother—who had helped arrange his earlier visit to the United States and a more recent trip to Saudi Arabia. Three additional diplomats of ambassadorial rank were posted to Washington just to work on the visit. This ambassador corps was assisted by some two dozen media specialists, including eleven public relations executives from leading Manila firms, who donated their services. In anticipation of the president's arrival, the embassy was refurbished and refurnished, and a constant stream of first- and second-level American military, congressional, and media personnel was entertained with meals prepared by a hotel chef and music provided by a

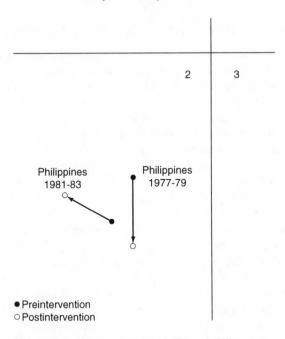

Figure 7.5. Effects of high- and low-visibility strategies: Philippines, 1977–79 and 1981–83

provincial song-and-dance group, all brought to Washington for this purpose.

In April, a Philippines exposition was presented at Bloomingdale's department store in New York, with Mrs. Marcos as the featured participant. Outdoor feasts were held for some 3,000 Filipino-Americans in the Washington area and some 12,000 in the San Francisco area; a government-subsidized Filipino restaurant was opened in Washington's Georgetown section in time for the official party to dine there during the visit; and a new English-language newspaper, the *Philippine Monitor,* commenced publication (Radcliffe, 1982; Lachica, 1982). This weekly newspaper was staffed by journalists at the Washington embassy, who filed their stories directly to Manila, where the paper was made up. Some 50,000 copies were then flown to the United States on the government-owned airline and distributed free of charge to the Filipino-American community (Radcliffe, 1982). To appreciate the real purpose of this effort, one must realize that this newspaper was added to a flow of Filipino-American communication that already included nineteen newspapers, eight newsletters or bulletins, and one magazine, at least thirteen of which could be classified as anti-Marcos (Hart, 1977).

In addition, the embassy's media relations group talked with some 170 American reporters, and shortly before Marcos's arrival, hundreds of journalists were presented with press kits in the form of expensive bamboo briefcases stuffed with promotional materials including a book, one of *seven* crimson-bound hardcover volumes, ostensibly written by Marcos and published just before his visit. Thousands of posters, T-shirts, and miniature Philippine flags were distributed; Washington was blanketed with signs proclaiming "Long Live Marcos and Reagan"; and hundreds of people were bused from as far away as Norfolk, Virginia, to participate in an unofficial welcoming ceremony at the Washington Monument, which was itself timed to correspond to prime television viewing hours in Manila, where it was broadcast live (Lachica, 1982; Rosellini, 1982).

Altogether, this effort was estimated to have cost some $5 million (National Public Radio, 1982). An embassy spokesman told the *Wall Street Journal* that this public relations blitz was intended to counter the "bad image" of Marcos and the Philippines in the U.S. press. "We have lost the public-opinion battle practically by default," he stated. "Nobody has made a sustained effort to tell our side of the story" (Lachica, 1982). Clearly such an effort was made in this instance.

The problem for the Filipinos was that the telling itself became the story. Articles about the campaign were published in the *New York Times,* the *Washington Post,* and the *Wall Street Journal,* and reporters at the time characterized the press kit, in particular, as the most elaborate they had ever seen. The net effect, as illustrated in Figure 7.5, was to raise the visibility of the Philippines in the news, but to make even more negative its portrayal.

One might interpret the comparative results of these two efforts as indicating that American public relations personnel are more capable than their Filipino counterparts, but that would miss the point. The problem here was threefold. First, the Filipinos were quite open about their efforts to manage the presidential image. Efforts at persuasive manipulation that are overt and easily recognized are also easily rejected. Second, whatever the costs of their lack of subterfuge, the Filipinos' effort failed as well on the basis of wretched excess. Even if theirs was a good effort for a good cause, it was badly overdone. But third, and most importantly, the Filipinos had the wrong strategy. In a situation that called for lowering the threshhold of public awareness of the Marcos visit, their entire effort was designed to "hype" the visit and raise visibility. And, as one might well expect, their failure appropriately to sense the image environment produced disastrous results.

Self-Interest Will Out: Iran

A similar fate befell a campaign waged in behalf of the shah's Iran in the mid-1970s, and for a related reason. In this instance, the public relations effort became not only visible to journalists and the U.S. public, but centrally involved in a domestic controversy. The observations cover the period from March 1974 through August 1976.

Iran began this period with an image in the south*east* quadrant of our typology, which is to say that its initial news image was positively valenced, but low in visibility. News coverage at the time focused on modernization efforts and economic development, cooperation with U.S. banks and defense firms, Iran's importance as a regional power and as an emerging force in world affairs, and its reliance on American military assistance. This was balanced somewhat by discussions of political prisoners, human rights, violations, and corruption, but such negative news was not dominant.

During the first fifteen months that we examined, the shah traveled widely, Secretary of State Kissinger visited Iran, the Iranian government granted a loan to Grumman Corporation and promised financial assistance to ailing Pan American Airways, several major U.S. banks and corporations began operations in the country, and in month 15 of the time series (June of 1975), the shah visited the United States.

In month 12, Iran (through its national airline) contracted with the first of two American public relations firms, Carl Byoir and Associates, for advice and counsel.[5] At about the same time, both events and news images turned for the worse. Northrup Corporation was implicated in a bribery scandal involving an Iranian prince, separate terrorist attacks took the lives of several American military and embassy officials, and Iran was forced to borrow money in international financial markets. At that point (month 18), Iran hired a second American public relations consultant, Ruder and Finn, to work on its image.

Over the next three months, little hard news of Iran appeared in the

New York Times, but there were articles about the development of urban centers, the major role to be played by U.S. corporations in the Iranian economy, the stability and continuity of the Iranian government, the development of an indigenous electronics industry, plans for a new medical center, the government's search for ways to end bribery, and the shah's plans to rebuild Xerxes' reception hall. In month 19, the shah granted an extensive personal interview to the *Times.* In month 22, the United States announced its intention to sell AWACS planes to Iran. The country was on a roll.

In January 1976 (month 23 in the series), the *New York Times* made public the fact that Marion Javits, wife of the U.S. senator from New York, who was a member of the committee on foreign relations, was employed by Ruder and Finn in its efforts in behalf of Iran. In fact, Mrs. Javits had apparently brought the contract, valued at over half a million dollars for one year, into the firm for what was to have been a $67,500 fee (Bender, 1976). In the weeks that followed, no fewer than fifteen articles about the public relations effort and the Javits connection appeared in the newspaper, all with a generally critical tone. Senator Javits, in particular, found the matter a profound embarrassment and pressured his wife into resigning from the account (Javits, 1981).

During this same period, Iran was once again forced to borrow funds, the Iranian military became involved in a war in Oman, the shah threatened to reduce purchases of U.S.-manufactured arms, and the United States ended its training of Iranian police forces. On March 15, 1976 (month 25), the shah directly threatened the United States, telling an interviewer from *U.S. News & World Report* that Iran "can hurt [the United States] as badly if not more so than you can hurt us" if the flow of American arms were cut. On March 25, Ruder and Finn terminated its contract to provide public relations services.

Figure 7.6 summarizes Iran's news image through this turbulent period. For purposes of illustration, the series is divided into three segments. The first (Iran 1) represents the months during which the Byoir contract was in effect, the second (Iran 2) those corresponding with the Ruder and Finn contract *before* the role of Marion Javits was made public, and the third (Iran 3) the months following disclosure of the Javits connection.

The image shift during the period of the Byoir contract clearly represents either an absence or a failure of image management. Iran 1 differs from most other countries discussed here in that its pretest image resided

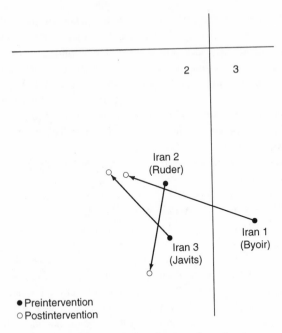

Figure 7.6. Public Relations intervention attracts controversy: Iran, 1974–76

east of the valence midpoint—it began the period with a positive image. The objective in such an instance, according to the present analysis, is enhancement and reinforcement of the existing image. Given the Iranian experience, however, one might conclude either that this strategy was not followed in this case, or that it was attempted without success.

In the event, the explanation may be quite straightforward. The public relations firm in question, Carl Byoir and Associates, had long been sensitive to criticism it received for having handled the German tourism account during the Hitler years and had been known to eschew overtly political work. Moreover, the contract in question was relatively small, amounting to some $50,000 plus expenses (Bender, 1976). It is thus quite possible that the firm defined its role in expressly nonpolitical terms, regardless of whether or not this matched the expectation of the Iranian government. In effect, then, the shift in the news image of Iran 1 was in no measure a product of the public relations effort. There was no experimental event.

The image shift associated with Iran 2 was consistent with our expectations in two ways. First, it demonstrated the typical three-month lag before changes were observed. Second, the changes themselves were consistent with the early stages of an image-management campaign beginning, as this one did, in the southwest quadrant, focusing primarily on a statistically significant reduction in visibility. The westward drift in valence was not significant. All of this ''progress,'' however, was offset by the Javits disclosure, as shown by the movement of Iran 3 back to significantly higher levels of visibility and negative valence. The controversy ended any opportunity Iran might have had to enhance its portrayal in the news.

The Power of History: South Africa and Southern Rhodesia

Finally, we compared the effects of public relations campaigns undertaken in behalf of the two white-ruled states of Southern Africa during the 1970s, South Africa and Southern Rhodesia, against the news-image effects of outbreaks of antiregime political violence that occured in each during that period.

Both countries were governed during the 1970s by white minority regimes, both had in place extensive government propaganda machines, and both contracted for the services of American public relations consultants to help improve their respective images and their political standing in the United States. But both, too, had politically active black majorities striving for power. In Southern Rhodesia, this striving took the form of a civil war that was overtly supported by the neighboring black states and at least indirectly backed by some Western governments. This civil war was characterized by a more or less constant level of conflict. In South Africa, violence was restricted to mass insurgency in several black areas, most notably Soweto, and was characteristically sporadic and unpredictable by comparison.

In the case of Southern Rhodesia, the public relations effort provided a defense against the external effects of the continuing and predictable domestic strife. During the year following the signing of the public relations contract the government engaged in a variety of seemingly image-related activities including, but not limited to, establishing an information office in Washington, conducting a press tour of a village that had recently been subjected to a guerrilla attack, portraying the ''kidnapping'' of black children by Botswana-based rebels, drawing attention to guerrilla raids on Catholic missions, and developing and publicizing "protected villages" for the black population. In addition, a rumor was circulated in the United States that white women throughout the country were contemplating suicide at the mere thought of majority rule.

In South Africa, though the expectation at the time of signing was probably much the same—the country was, at the time, free of violence, but had a very negative image abroad—the context of the image-enhancement effort rapidly developed in a different direction. Just as the campaign was being implemented, South Africa was struck by a wave of uprisings originating in Soweto. This violence, and the government response that followed, presented a crisis in the image environment that could hardly have been anticipated. What had been a stable, if generally negative, news image was suddenly destabilized.

Figure 7.7 summarizes the changes in news portrayals of South Af-

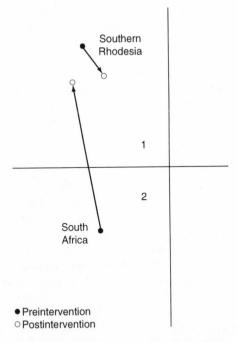

Figure 7.7. Violence as a countermeasure to Public Relations: South Africa and Southern Rhodesia, 1975–77

rica and Southern Rhodesia during this period. The figure shows a very slight improvement in the image of Southern Rhodesia associated in time with the public relations effort, this despite the historical forces working in the opposite direction. South Africa's image, however, worsened dramatically. In analyzing these data, we were able to separate to some extent the impact on news portrayals of the public relations effort and the extant political violence. This analysis led us to conclude that, in actuality, the public relations activity had had a salutary effect on the valence dimension of *both* sets of images. Without its campaign to control the external dissemination of images of violence, Southern Rhodesia's image would have been considerably more negative. And even in South Africa, the image-enhancement effort conveyed a more positive image of that country than would otherwise have been the case. For all of that, however, the public relations consultants could not, on balance, overcome the force of historical reality.

Conclusion

Our examination of the impact of public relations efforts on news portrayals of those countries that engage in strategic public diplomacy, then, have led us to four conclusions. First, as we had predicted, there do exist consistencies in the timing and direction of image changes associated with public relations activities of the sort described here. And second, under normal circumstances, these activities can have a significant impact on the images of foreign nations that are presented to the U.S. public. Taken together, these two points define the range of what is strategically viable in the management of national images. But third, when circumstances vary from normality in ways that place the image-enhancement effort itself on the media and public agendas—when the consultants or their activities go public—institutional and psychological defenses may be raised, and the likelihood of success is markedly reduced. And finally, even the most effective public relations effort is unlikely to possess the power to overcome substantial historical forces once they have been set in motion against the interests of the client. These latter points define the operational limits that constrain would-be persuaders.

8

Agenda Dynamics and External Influence on U.S. Foreign Policymaking

As we noted in Chapter 7, one of the most influential theories of political communication in recent years has been the theory of agenda setting, first stated by McCombs and Shaw (1972), with its concentration on the linkage between media content and public opinion and its argument that public attention will, over time, be channeled to those issues or actors who receive disproportionate attention in the media. The notion of agenda setting offers an appropriate starting point for our development of a conceptual framework with which to illuminate the practice of strategic public diplomacy, in part because it deals with two key elements of the public diplomatist's art—the media and the public—but also because one of its central tenets—that the media ''tell'' people not what to think, but what to think *about*—was first set forth by Bernard Cohen in his 1963 treatise on the influence of media on the making of foreign policy.

Agenda Setting as a Theoretical Construct

As a theory, agenda setting has several important assets. First, the concept itself is both intuitively obvious and appealing. It simply seems to make sense. Second, it suggests a straightforward inventory of independent and dependent variables, offers some fairly explicit predictions regarding the relationships among these, and provides a parsimonious explanation for those associations that are, in fact, observed. Third, and directly as a product of the first two points, agenda setting has suggested to literally hundreds of scholars a cluster of manageable research projects by which the theory might be tested and has provided a legitimized rationale for soliciting research support. Fourth, the elements of agenda-setting research display an evident correspondence to readily observable real-world phenomena and the products of that research have equally evident real-world application. And fifth, the timing of the development of agenda setting was especially fortuitous, coming as it did when other avenues of political communication inquiry seemed to have turned into blind alleys, but when media- and other communication-related phenomena were of unmistakeable and seemingly increasing political significance. As a result of these factors, research in the agenda-setting tradition, and, therefore, the influence of the theory itself, has proliferated.

Set against these strengths, however, is one important liability that became evident only with the passage of time and the development of a body of research in the agenda-setting tradition. For, as much research as we have devoted to agenda-setting phenomena and as much as we have learned about them—and both categories are quite large—what we have really learned is how narrow this conceptual framework is. Whether in Shaw and McCombs's early characterization of the approach—"[a]genda-setting asserts that audiences learn [the relative] saliences [of various stories] from the news media, incorporating a similar set of weights into their personal agendas. . . . [T]hese saliences . . . are among the most important message attributes transmitted to the audience" (1977: 11)—or in more recent formulations, it has become clear in the light of the two decades of subsequent research in political communication that agenda-related phenomena are both broader in scope and more significant than the extant formulation of this theory could accommodate.

What this suggests is the presence of a "levels of theory" problem. In its time, agenda setting was a relatively general theory. Although grounded in the election related and voting behavior related paradigm that dominated the study of political behavior in the 1960s and early 1970s—indeed, except for the serendipitous enterprise of an unnamed editor of *Public Opinion Quarterly*, who retitled the initial McCombs and Shaw manuscript "The Agenda-Setting Function of Mass Media," the piece would have carried a title on the order of "Media Coverage of Elections in a Small Southern Town," and the academic industry constructed around the notion of agenda setting might never have laid its first brick (Shaw, 1992)—agenda setting pointed the way to a more generic and comprehensive understanding of political communication processes, so that today, though much research in this tradition still focuses on voters and election campaigns, substantial work has looked as well at issue development, media influence, and policy effects that go well beyond a simple electoral context. In doing so, however, much of this literature has outpaced the conceptual framework on which it purports to be based. Our research, in other words, has gotten out in front of our theory.

Agenda Dynamics as an Alternative Construct

It was with this in mind that I proposed a few years ago (Manheim, 1987) what I termed a "model of agenda dynamics," a formulation whose objective was (and remains) to integrate several apparently diverse lines of political communication inquiry into one logical whole, the better to examine the relationships among both the several conceptual frameworks themselves and the phenomena to which they relate. In the balance of this chapter, I will delineate the model in some detail.

The central notion of agenda dynamics is that much of what we have defined as political communication occurs within a comprehensive system of interactive agendas. Principal among these are the by-now-familiar agendas of the media, the public, and the policymakers. The media agenda comprises those issues, actors, events, images, and viewpoints that receive time or space in publications or broadcasts that are available to a given audience at a given time. Similarly, the public agenda comprises those items which are the subject of public attention, whether at the individual or the aggregate level, at a given time. And the policy agenda, in the words of Cobb, Ross, and Ross (1976: 126) is "the list of items which decision makers have formally accepted for serious consideration."

Agenda dynamics suggests that each of these agendas, drawing as it does on a distinct set of political actors, institutions, and processes, has its own internal dynamic, for example, media economics and newsroom decision making in the first instance, the sociological and cognitive processing of information in the second, and organizational pressures and constraints in the third. These and other factors have been explored in the literatures of several disciplines. In addition, like the related

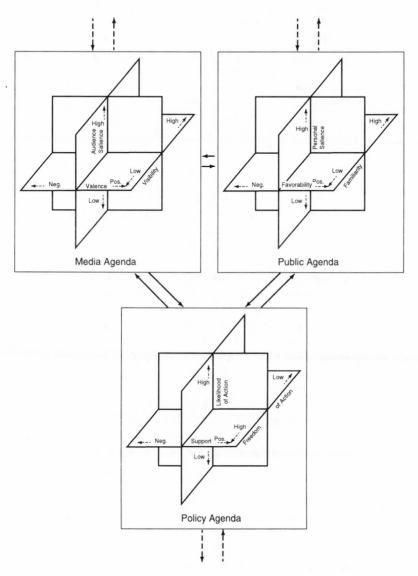

Figure 8.1. A model of agenda dynamics

concepts of agenda setting and agenda building, agenda dynamics recognizes that these various agendas interact with one another across a network of informational, institutional, and behavioral bridges.

These internal and interactive characteristics are summarized in Figure 8.1, which identifies some key attributes of the information that is arrayed on each agenda. The model illustrated in the figure, I should note, is not intended to constitute a complete statement of the agenda dynamics framework, but represents instead one possible statement of an agenda dynamics *approach* to understanding a large class of phenomena. Thus it is the *idea* of the dimensions specified in the model, at least as much as their specification, that is of central concern.

The Media Agenda

Each component agenda represented in Figure 8.1 has been characterized as comprising three dimensions. With respect to the media agenda, these include visibility, audience salience, and valence. *Visibility* refers to the amount and/or prominence of coverage afforded by the media to any actor, event, or object. Research over several decades has shown that such factors as story location, the number of insertions, the size of headlines, and the use of graphics affect the amount of attention an audience will devote to one or another topic in the news (Behr and Iyengar, 1985; Greenberg and Garfinkle, 1963; Hvistendahl, 1968; Mehling, 1959; Powers and Kearl, 1968; Williams and Semlak, 1978). In our present terms, this means that topics that are relatively more visible in the media are more likely than others to be transfered to the public agenda.

Audience salience refers to the stated or implied relevance of news content to audience needs. Salience cues might include references to such factors as social stability, economic security, or the general well-being or preference structures of the audience. A principal product of the reconstituting of news in both the broadcast and the print media over the last twenty years or so (Bennett, 1988b) for the purpose of maximizing audience share and the net revenue generated for media corporations by news has been the greater emphasis on points of psychological contact among the audience, the news providers, and the news events themselves. In many cases today, news items are selected and molded to make such connections in the expectation that an audience that is personally involved in processing such information will be both larger and more loyal to the news medium than might otherwise be the case. At a more conceptual level, the function of such symbolic linkages between the news and the audience is to integrate news content with existing cognitions (Graber, 1988) and to enhance the perceived importance of news content among members of the public.

The third dimension of the media agenda, *valence,* refers to the general sense of favor, neutrality, or disfavor associated with the portrayal of a given object. Here, too, the proposed model varies from the initial statement of agenda setting, which held, in part, that the media do not tell people "what to think." I am not arguing the converse, but would suggest that messages are wrapped in cues that convey judgments about objects in the news, and that audiences are not insensitive to these cues.

The Public Agenda

With respect to the public agenda, the principal dimensions include familiarity, or the degree of public awareness of, or attention to, a given attitude object; personal salience, or the internalization of the linkage between events in the news and one's personal needs or self-interest; and favorability, or a summary affective judgment about the topic or object in question.

Familiarity with an issue, actor, or event has been a central focus in studies of agenda setting from the outset (see, e.g., Gantz, Trenholm, and Pittman, 1976; Kent and Rush, 1976), but has not always been treated as an analytically distinct phenomenon. More often than not, the dependent variables in agenda-setting research have been defined as levels of public concern with or about an issue, a construction that fails to distinguish clearly between affects and cognitions. Indeed, in a basic formulation of the theory itself, Shaw and McCombs (1977) describe agenda setting as a cognition-based phenomenon (p. 7), then immediately and for the balance of their analysis turn their attention to the salience rather than the cognitive content of issues (pp. 7–8 passim). Subsequent research (for example, Erbring, Goldenberg, and Miller, 1980; Graber, 1988) has made clear, however, the utility of establishing a distinction between familiarity and salience, between what people think about, on the one hand, and how important they think it is, or how they think it is important, on the other.

In one form or another, *salience* has long been recognized as an important component of public opinion (for early examples, see Czudnowski, 1968; Jennings and Zeigler, 1970; Lane and Sears, 1964; Verba and Nie, 1972). More recent studies (Behr and Iyengar, 1985; Einsiedel, Salomone, and Schneider, 1984; Lang and Lang, 1981) have weighed media effects against those of personal experience in assessing agenda setting. A common element in all of these and other related studies is the recognition that the susceptibility of individuals to influence is in some measure dependent on the personal importance that they attach to incoming information and to the existing affects or cognitions with which it might interact.

The third dimension of the public agenda is *favorability,* the expressed preference of an individual or a public (depending on one's level of analysis) with respect to a given agenda item. Though there is relatively little evidence to demonstrate agenda-setting effects on favorability comparable to those on familiarity or salience (an exception is Page, Shapiro, and Dempsey, 1985), perhaps because the formulation of the theory explicitly negated these effects and discouraged related inquiry, such preferences are very much a part of public opinion and an evident target of systematic attempts to influence that opinion. Indeed, Kotler (1982: 56–62) characterizes political marketing in precisely these terms.

The Policy Agenda

Downs (1972), Cobb and Elder (1972), Cook and King (1982), and Kingdon (1984), among others, have characterized the ways in which issues move—or are moved—on and off the policy agenda. Two central themes in these and related studies are (1) the likelihood that a governmental body will act on a given issue or respond to a given actor or event, and (2) the substantive nature of any policy decision or action that may emerge. In the present instance, these dimensions have been labeled *likelihood of action* and *degree of support.* The latter characterizes action as more or less in accord with the policy objectives or the political standing of a given issue position or actor. The third dimension of the policy agenda represented in Figure 8.1 is *freedom of action,* a concept that derives largely from the work of Murray Edelman (especially 1964, 1971, and 1988), in which it is argued that the degree of freedom of action available to policymakers will vary directly with the level of quiescence of the citizenry. The present analysis extends the same argument to specific agenda items.

Value of the Agenda-Dynamics Approach

Studies within the agenda-setting tradition, then, as well as others with findings of relevance, have established a firm base of knowledge regarding behaviors within and among the media, public, and policymakers. What the notion of agenda dynamics adds to this mix is twofold. First, agenda dynamics suggests that the internal dynamics of each agenda both influence and are influenced by the linkages that agenda has with the others in the system. Although this point may seem intuitively obvious, it has been neither stated nor integrated into analyses of agenda-related phenomena to date. Second, agenda dynamics points toward some of the ways in which internal dynamics and interagenda linkages might interact. This is accomplished in large measure through a typology of agenda-related hypotheses, which is summarized in Table 8.1.

A growing body of recent research speaks in much the same terms as the agenda dynamics model we have developed here. Examples include Adams (1987); Bolce, DeMaio, and Muzzio (1987); Green and Gerken (1989); Harrington (1989); Iyengar (1990); Krosnick (1990); Margolis and Mauser (1989); Modigliani and Modigliani (1987); Rowland and Payne (1987); and Salwen (1988). For these studies, agenda dynamics suggests a logic by which such notions as salience and visibility can "travel" from one agenda to another. Other studies employ concepts and variables that are not specified in the model as presented here, but that do fit well with our more general focus on the interaction between the internal dynamics of each agenda and its exchanges with the others. Thus research by John Mueller (1988), Keith Mueller (1988), and Erfle, McMillan, and Grofman (1990), all of whom deal in part with the role of perceived threat, and Green and Guth (1989), who suggest the importance of segmentation within the public agenda, can be seen as suggesting alternative formulations of the principal dimensions of various agendas while confirming the utility of the larger linkage between internal dynamics and interagenda exchange.

At a more practical level, agenda dynamics offers a means of accommodating assumptions that are made in the literature, but which exceed the bounds of current theory. A prime case in point is the use of the term "agenda setting" in discussions of media or public impacts on the policy agenda, or public and policymaker impacts on the media agenda (for example, Keith Mueller, 1988; Leff, Protess, and Brooks, 1986; Pritchard, 1986; and Berkowitz, 1987). The processes described in these

Table 8.1. A Typology of Agenda-Related Hypotheses

Type A: Hypotheses relating to the initial location (attributes) of an item on a single agenda

---

A.1. Location on the media agenda
   IV: events; characteristics and operation of media decision making; efforts to influence that decision making
   DV: attributes of items on the media agenda; temporal patterns of development
A.2. Location on the public agenda
   IV: events; source and content of available information regarding new issues (e.g., mediated versus experiential knowledge)
   DV: attributes of items on the public agenda; temporal patterns of development
A.3. Location on the policy agenda
   IV: events; development of new knowledge or expertise; changes in personnel; political processes
   DV: attributes of items on the policy agenda; temporal patterns of development

---

Type B: Hypotheses relating to change in the location (attributes) of an item on a single agenda

---

B.1. Change in location on the media agenda
   IV: events; editorial decisions; maturation processes affecting actors or events; external efforts at manipulation of existing images; changing definitions or interpretations of journalistic norms
   DV: changes in attributes of items on the media agenda; temporal patterns of change; susceptibility or resistance to change
B.2. Change in location on the public agenda
   IV: events; changes in underlying context of public opinion; changes in sources of information (e.g., their number or diversity); political socialization; maturation processes affecting actors or events
   DV: changes in attributes of items on the public agenda; temporal patterns of change; susceptibility or resistance to change; reinterpretation of existing images or perceptions (reorganization of schema)

Type B: Hypotheses relating to change in the location (attributes) of an item on a single agenda

---

B.3. Change in location on the policy agenda
   IV: events; new or accumulating knowledge or information; changes in relative influence of political actors; changes in personnel occupying policymaking positions; maturation processes affecting actors or events
   DV: changes in attributes of items on the policy agenda; temporal patterns of change; susceptibility or resistance to change

continued

Table 8.1. A Typology of Agenda-Related Hypotheses (*continued*)

Type C: Hypotheses relating to the movement of a given item from one agenda to another

---

C.1. Media-public exchanges
- IV: audience preferences or behaviors; events; initial attributes of the item; specificity or obtrusiveness of issues; economic motivations of media organizations
- DV: interactive locational effects (those relating initial positioning in the dimensioned space of one agenda to subsequent positioning in the dimensioned space of another); direction of exchanges (e.g., recursiveness); temporal characteristics of exchanges

C.2. Media-policy exchanges
- IV: patterns of media use by policymakers; newsmaking and newsgathering behaviors; regulatory policies
- DV: interactive locational effects; direction of exchanges; temporal characteristics of exchanges

C.3. Public-policy exchanges
- IV: changes in public opinion polls on a given issue; proximity or results of elections; public education or persuasion activities by policy actors; differential characteristics of issue publics
- DV: interactive locational effects; direction of exchanges; temporal characteristics of exchanges

---

Type D: Hypotheses relating to the development pattern of specific issues or images, or of general classes of issues or images

---

- IV: specificity, obtrusiveness, instrumentality, or other characteristics of issues
- DV: specific operations of the overall process of agenda dynamics from initiation of an issue through policy action (and, for iterative processes, beyond)

Source: Derived from Table 22.1 in Manheim (1987: 510–13). The original table incorporates additional literature citations as well as specific examples of hypotheses falling within each class.

studies and others like them do amount to something that is functionally equivalent to agenda setting, but at the level of explanation, they are not consistent with the concept as originally formulated and applied. The ideas expressed in this research are good ones—the point is only that the terminology we use to describe them must catch up with the concepts. The framework provided by agenda dynamics accomplishes that purpose.

9

The Evolution of Influence

In 1622, when Pope Gregory XV established what he termed the Congregatio de Propaganda Fide, an arm of the Catholic church whose objective was to spread the faith among non-Christians, he institutionalized, arguably for the first time, what was even then an emerging science of influence. As our examples in Chapter 1 suggest, political leaders had long appreciated the value of a carefully crafted image. And Machiavelli, writing a full century earlier, had delineated the advantages of adopting a comprehensive and empirically grounded communication *strategy*. But it was not until technique was married to organization that the ground was prepared for the emergence of persuasive and manipulative communication as an instrument of effective political action. Even then, it took more than three additional centuries for the science of influence to mature.

I have explored elsewhere (Manheim, 1991a) the contemporary practice of strategic political communication and have argued that its effects on our society are both pervasive and deleterious. In the present instance, I take that argument as a given. The purpose here has been to examine in rather greater detail a particular subset of efforts at influence through communication, those in which actors who are (mostly) external to the American political scene introduce elements of strategy into their U.S.-directed campaigns of public diplomacy for the wholly intertwined purposes of improving the setting in which foreign policy decisions of interest to them are made, and of stimulating or deterring such decision making.

The use of strategic communication in this particular context presents us with two sets of issues that, on the basis of the evidence presented here, I find compelling. The first are the *political issues,* which revolve around the proprieties and utilities of permitting, or even encouraging, other nations, relatively unimpeded, to gain access to the domestic political processes that generate ideas and support for U.S. foreign policy. The second are the *conceptual issues,* which contribute to a comprehensive understanding of how and why communication strategies are effective and to a perspective on the much larger conflict between basic and applied uses of social scientific knowledge. In this final chapter I will delineate some of the issues on both agendas and will, in the process, consider one of their most salient traits, their interdependence.

The Political Questions

In some ways, the political questions associated with the practice of strategic public diplomacy are most vital because they revolve so closely around the defining issue of freedom of speech and the responsibility that accompanies its exercise. Among these are the control of communication technologies (in this instance, *social* technologies), ethical conduct and disclosure, self-interest and the public interest, and the structuring of the policymaking environment. I shall outline each set of issues in its turn.

Control of Communication Technologies

A consistent argument in these pages has been that communication strategies of the sort employed in contemporary American politics, and increasingly in U.S.-directed public diplomacy, are grounded in a newly emergent social technology[1] that draws on an ever-widening base of knowledge, derived from conceptual developments in such fields as political science and social psychology, and supported by the voluminous product of what are now generations of survey research, focus-group data, organizational studies, content analyses, and the like. An ironic element of this development is that, though much of the underlying science has been paid for by government through the National Science Foundation and other granting agencies and though much of the technology has long been available to the U.S. government to use for its own international purposes, it appears to be the leasing out of this knowledge by the U.S. private sector, rather than its application by the public sector, that is predominant. Aside from an early mention, we have not considered here the use (or absence of use) of strategic communication in the conduct of public diplomacy by the United States, and my unsubstantiated assertion that it is, by comparison, relatively ineffective is, for the moment, just that. That is necessarily a subject to be reserved for another opus. But we have, I think, demonstrated the purposefulness and the effectiveness of such efforts targeted closer to home, and it is worthwhile to search out the origins of such action.

In Chapter 2, we examined the coming of age of the half-billion-dollar-a-year industry that has emerged to represent foreign interests in the United States. In particular, in Table 2.1, we saw evidence of strong and sustained growth in both the number of firms providing services and the number of new foreign principals year to year. One question we did not address in the related discussion, however, was that of the proverbial chicken and egg. That is, which came first, the industry or the clients? It is not a trivial question.

Figure 9.1 presents the data on two indicators from Table 2.1 in graphic form. The first is the number of firms registered with the Department of Justice as foreign agents for each year from 1967 through 1986. The second is the number of new foreign principals with whom such contracts are signed, in this instance covering the period 1971 through 1987. The trend in both instances is, not surprisingly, upward. More interesting, however, is the timing of the respective movements. The figure suggests very clearly that industry growth *preceded* growth in the client base. In other words, the supply of service providers grew, and grew rapidly, before the demand for their services was in place. This means that in order to assure their economic viability, the purveyors of these services have had to market them aggressively to prospective clients. And in that process, they have had to educate prospective clients as to their value. That is to say, because strategic communication is potentially both innovative and expensive, would-be agents of foreign interests have needed to communicate to their clientele a sense of what they were doing and of the underlying rational for doing it. Governments and others will want to understand as fully as possible the benefits they will derive before they will spend the sums of money required to sustain so large an industry. We saw evidence of such a dynamic, for example, in the relationship between Hill and Knowlton and the Citizens for a

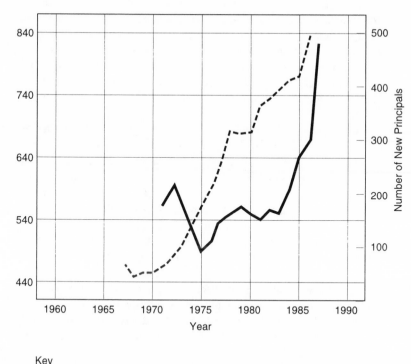

Figure 9.1. Number of registered firms and new foreign principals: 1967–87

Free Kuwait, particularly at the time when a change in the thematic emphasis of the public relations effort was proposed.

It is important to remember that we are dealing here not with some electronic device or piece of hardware whose function can be isolated, more or less completely, from the technique of its creation, but with elements of social technology where such separation is difficult, if not impossible, to achieve. Thus, strategic communicators in the employ of foreign interests are exporters, not merely of the services they purvey, but of the underlying intellectual property on which their industry is based. Bit by bit, they are conveying knowledge about the techniques of strategic communication to clients as they attract and serve them.

As this trend continues for some period, a number of foreign entities will inevitably acquire a broader base of sophisticated knowledge about the operations of the U.S. political system. As a result, they will acquire as well the ability, *operating outside of the current structure of regulatory oversight,* to conduct strategic public diplomacy in their own behalf with greater effect than they are presently able to do so and without their current degree of dependency on domestically grounded service providers.

This has at least two implications. First, it suggests that over time the services provided by the industry, at least to its most sophisticated clients, will evolve away from consulting on technique and toward the marketing of narrower forms of expertise focused on peculiarities of the contemporaneous American scene. In effect, the industry will have exported its intellectual capital in much the same way that the automobile industry has its production capacity and will be left to focus on design and marketing for the unique aspects of the American market. Second, the making of foreign policy in the United States will become increasingly subject to subtle but effective influence from interested outside parties. We will, in essence, become captives of our long-standing commitment to a free international flow of information, and in ways that are, ironically, not unlike those to which nations of the Third World have so long objected. That the technology was homegrown will not make the tomato taste sweeter.

Ethical Conduct and Disclosure

There is a stigma that attaches to the term ''foreign agent,'' one made all the more onerous by the campaign waged by H. Ross Perot, Pat Choate, and others to limit the representation of foreign interests in U.S. policymaking. And yet, on inspection, there can be little doubt of the patriotism of virtually all who register to provide such services. They see foreign agentry as a wholly legitimate enterprise—indeed, it is for many merely an extension of a line of business that they also provide to corporate, partisan, and other domestic clients—and as an opportunity to encourage open and balanced debate on important policy questions. It is an exercise of their own free speech and an extension of the right to speak to others whose voices might otherwise not be heard.

It may or may not be the case that foreign governments, foreign-owned corporations, and other such entities have a claim on the protections of the First Amendment. That is a legal question and one to be resolved by constitutional lawyers and jurists. But it does seem fair to hold that whatever the rights of these entities may be and however broadly defined, the government and people of the United States have a compelling public interest in knowing who is speaking. That is a political question and one to be resolved by the people through their representatives in the media and the government.

For its part, Congress has an obligation to develop for itself and for the public a much better understanding of the process and effects of strategic public diplomacy. Attempts, like that of Congressman Glickman as described in note 1 to Chapter 2, to fine tune the registration process are functional, but they are superficial. They will help to assure that information about foreign representational activity is entered into the public record more extensively than is the case at present, but they do not address in any way the *trade* issues associated with the operations of this industry—such as the transfer of strategically sensitive social technology—and they provide no protection whatever from direct interventions by foreign interests that are not covered by the registration concept.

There are, obviously, important First Amendment interests here that must be protected. But, as I hope will be clear from the analysis in this book, there are important, but little-recognized, *strategic* interests at stake as well. They revolve around the question: how free is the *process* of making U.S. foreign policy to pursue and protect *American* interests? I would suggest that the answer is: not nearly as free and independent as we like to think. We live in an interdependent world. There is not, cannot be, and should not be an ability on the part of any nation, including the United States, to make foreign policy in a vacuum. But, by the same token, there is not, cannot be, and should not be any excuse for ignoring or underestimating the effects of the concerted efforts made by interested external parties to influence the policy process. That argument can only be strengthened by the realization that the technology of influence is our own.

Precisely because of the free speech issues and the need in a democratic society to tolerate a wide range of expression, defined not only by point of view but by point of origin, the resolution of these issues cannot be left to government alone. For as we have seen, though they may have governmental actors as secondary target, many of the activities of strategic communicators are designed to treat journalists and news organizations as primary targets of opportunity. As a result, journalists are on the firing line. And as it happens, they are also especially well equipped, if so inclined, to focus public attention on efforts at manipulation. For journalists are the principal consumers of the public record, a record that includes a great deal of information on the activities in question.

We know from the analysis in Chapter 7 that such a focusing of attention can mitigate the effects of efforts that are, prospectively, of marginal legitimacy, or none whatsoever. But we also know that, except in the most controversial of cases, journalists are disinclined to bring it about. One justification that is often offered by journalists, at least many with whom I have spoken over the years, for their lack of attention to international public relations efforts is their casual assumption that such efforts are ineffective. I hope that the weight of argument in this book will suggest that this is simply incorrect. To the contrary, the techniques that are employed are often far more subtle and sophisticated than the journalists tend to assume, and their impact is potentially substantial.

Another justification frequently offered for journalistic inattention to image-management efforts is the demonstrable lack of audience attention to foreign affairs news, which is, in fact, one of the central facilitating realities of the campaigns themselves. Yet it seems to me that because of their other characteristics—conflict, drama, high stakes, and so forth—some of these efforts are sufficiently newsworthy in and of themselves to merit more coverage and may even provide a mechanism through which greater public interest in international affairs could be generated.

Finally, news organizations like to argue that they do not make the news, they merely report it. There is much in the literature of media research to suggest that this is an unduly, and perhaps purposefully, naive view of the world. But in this particular instance, we need not even draw breath from such arguments to make the point. For in this instance, the media are often targeted, and their behaviors are influenced, by image managers. Sometimes they are unaware of this. They have an affirmative obligation to minimize the number of such times. And when they are aware of it, they have an affirmative obligation publically to so note. In fairness, major national news media have given a bit more time and space to foreign agentry in recent years. But it is not yet enough.

Self-Interest and the Public Interest

Much of our discussion of industry and free speech issues to this point has been concerned with the relationship between the interests of the service providers and those of the public. The two are not mutually exclusive. For, if the public has an interest in receiving the views of foreign entities, and if those entities have some measure of rights to express their views and to attempt to influence policymaking to their advantage, the representation industry serves the public interest by facilitating such expression even as it serves its self-interest by profiting from doing so.

A special situation arises, however, when foreign agents are in a position to use the governmental equivalent of inside information on behalf of outside interests. This is the case, for instance, when federal officials with foreign trade or foreign policy responsibilities walk through the revolving door into the foreign interest representation industry. They become, in Choate's term, especially potent "agents of influence." A 1992 report to Congress (United States General Accounting Office, 1992) identified eighty-two former high-level federal officials—among them two senators, one member of the House of Representatives, seven White House officials, thirty-three senior congressional staff members, and thirty-nine officials of executive agencies—who left government between 1986 and 1991 and later represented foreign interests before the U.S. government. In the aggregate, they represented interests from forty-three countries.

Among the more prominent persons on this list were Mark Andrews, Don Bonker, William Brock, Paul Laxalt, and Mari Maseng. Perhaps more revealing, among the government job titles on the list were: deputy attorney general; staff director, Senate Foreign Relations Committee; special assistant to the president for legislative affairs; secretary of labor; director of policy, planning and analysis, Department of Energy; assistant secretary of commerce for international economic policy; assistant secretary of state for legislative affairs; ambassador, Office of the U.S. Trade Representative (also the chief of staff, an economist, and an assistant trade representative from the same agency); assistant secretary of commerce for trade development; staff director, Senate Select Committee on Intelligence; chief of staff, Office of the House Republican Leader; deputy under-secretary of the army; deputy secretary, Department of Energy; director of communications, the White House; executive director, House Budget Committee; director of international economic affairs, National Security Council; vice president and general counsel, Overseas Private Investment Council; deputy assistant to the president for national security; commissioner of customs; and counsel to the president. It is, in truth, an impressive inventory of expertise.

Only a modest proportion of the work undertaken by these refugees from public service could be classified as strategic public diplomacy, though a good deal more clearly takes the form of lobbying. And there are in place, in any event, postemployment conflict-of-interest statutes that restrict this activity in some important ways. Specifically, former officials are precluded from lobbying their old agencies or from lobbying on issues they managed, for periods of time varying from one year after departure to life. And the GAO report neither sought nor found any evidence that these laws were violated. But there are larger questions of propriety and the limits of entrepreneurship that should be addressed, questions that focus less on specific policy questions or lobbying activities than on our making available to foreign, and at least potentially contrary, interests in such degree the breadth of experience and perspective on both classes of issues and the governmental process per se through a device that is clearly and unambiguously driven by the self-interest of this subset of foreign agents.

The Policymaking Environment

Finally with respect to the political agenda, we ought to realize that the issues here relate directly to the quality of political dialogue and of information gathering that underlie our foreign policymaking. We can take a step in this direction by recognizing that, to a growing extent, the speech issues here are not solely those that revolve around freedom of expression, for it is often not unhindered *expression* that is the objective of strategic public diplomacy. Rather, it is *manipulation,* manipulation that can take the form of the suppression, or at least, the explicit discouragement of open debate, the harnessing of otherwise independent organizational imperatives, and the strategic management of information flows. *It is activity whose objective is sometimes less the freedom than the **structuring** of expression.* That is the aspect of strategic public diplomacy that most threatens the vitality of the political process, that must be more clearly recognized and understood, and from which the process must be more effectively protected.

The Conceptual Questions

The centrality of an enhanced understanding of the dangers that accompany the unfettered practice *upon* a society of strategic public diplomacy provides a natural bridge to the identification of important questions relating to the conceptual grounding of these same practices. These, I think, fall into two categories.

Enlightening the Scholarly Literature

The first of these categories focuses on the directions in which academic inquiry on questions related to foreign policy has developed and on new paths it might constructively follow.

I must confess here to being, by both training and inclination, what my colleagues in political science refer to as an "Americanist." That is, my background is in the study of American politics rather than international affairs or comparative analysis, and my interest is less in the workings of the international system per se than in the impact that such workings can have in the domestic arena. In the present context, this is at once a curse and a blessing. It is a curse because I cannot claim to be sufficiently widely read in the scholarly literatures of international relations, foreign policy studies, diplomatic practice, and the like to provide a reliable and comprehensive general characterization of the work found there. I am, instead, a selective reader. As a result, I operate from what I am certain is a less than representative sense of the balance of scholarly attention. For all of that, however, based on my fragmented reading of that literature, and more emphatically on conversations over the years with others who are indeed expert in the field and who tend to reinforce my prejudices, I would assert that those who do specialize in such inquiry tend to give far less than appropriate weight to the domestic politics of foreign policymaking, and especially to the impact on domestic politics of the sort of systematic campaigns of influence that I have detailed here. And yet, demonstrably now, these are real and significant phenomena. It is my belief, then, that studies of foreign policymaking that exclude such considerations are more or less seriously flawed, the degree being a function of the level of strategic communication activity present in the environment of any extant case.

In simplest terms, the issue is one of recognizing potentially salient independent, dependent, and intervening variables. For the reasons stated in Chapter 7, third-party interventions are regular features of the foreign policy process. Indeed, although the research reported here treated them as experimental events in a series of case studies, their number and regularity, as indicated in the industry analysis in Chapter 2, are sufficient that their presence or absence, or some characterization thereof, could be a valuable factor in explaining entire classes of foreign policy outcomes if these were merely reconceptualized as products of the domestic political process.

One counterargument to this view is that although popular reaction may affect the implementation of foreign policy once it is established, the policy itself is most likely a product of external geopolitical or other considerations. This, however, is more often assumed than demonstrated, and we have a growing catechism of examples that suggest otherwise. Moreover, it is important to realize that implementation of a foreign policy—or more to the point, the creation of a political environment in which it can be implemented—is an equally important focus of inquiry.

The agenda-dynamics model suggests numerous variables of demonstrated general significance that can reasonably be expected to operate in the making of U.S. foreign policy. They include aspects of media behavior, public perception and behavior, organizational and governmental behavior, and message construction. But most on point, they include as well a recognition at the level of theory development of the need to accommodate the target-country domestic *political* actions of diverse international participants. If these actions were regarded by the players themselves as irrelevant to the game, they would not spend an aggregated half billion dollars every year to engage in them. That alone makes them worthy of attention. But more than that, the substantial grounding in empirical social science that has, in fact, *created* these phenomena makes their inclusion in studies of foreign policymaking intellectually imperative. Such a communication-based perspective will not replace other, more established explanatory frameworks applied by scholars to further our understanding of this field, but it does have the potential to enhance the knowledge base in important ways. This is a lesson Bernard

Cohen (1963, 1973) proferred decades ago, and it is a lesson for our times today.

And that, I think, is where the blessing of the Americanist's perspective comes into play. For it is, as Cohen so rightly recognized, the American polity that produces policy options and political movement toward or away from them, whether in the area of foreign affairs or elsewhere. It follows that, to the extent that domestic considerations come into play, explanatory variables that structure those considerations must be incorporated into our analytical world view as well. And that brings us, in a sense, full circle. For just as strategic communication phenomena have come to play a central role in the American political process generally (Manheim, 1991a), they have gained greater and greater acceptance as loci of explanation in related scholarship, a fact that, as we have seen, itself traces to an idea spun off by Professor Cohen. Indeed, communication-grounded research now appears in numerous academic venues of political science analysis, and organizations of scholars pursuing such questions are thriving. Foreign policy studies can benefit from this trend.

Basic Versus Applied Social Research

The irony here, of course, is that social science research is failing to take adequately into account a phenomenon that owes its very existence to that very same body of research. For strategic political communication, whether in its public diplomacy guise or any other, is at heart a research-defined and a research-driven enterprise. Indeed, that is what separates it from the more touchy-feely artistry of the publicist. It is, as we said at the outset, an applied science of human behavior.

Perhaps the critical word in that last phrase is "applied." For the practitioners of strategic communication operate very much in the mode of the applied scientist, one who uses the tools of (social) inquiry to address and resolve specific problems with which she or he is presented. How better could we characterize the Wirthlin focus group that measured responses to Gulf conflict images than that? Academic researchers, on the other hand, are generally more accustomed to operating in the sphere of basic research, that which is devoted to more abstract exercises in concept building and theory development without substantial attention being devoted to concrete problem solving. Still, once we have identified a general phenomenon of demonstrated practical significance, why would it not be incorporated into these more basic explanatory efforts?

Perhaps the answer lies in the relative youthfulness of social scientific inquiry, which in practical terms is arguably a phenomenon of the twentieth century alone. In that sense, it may be that we are observing the collective professional equivalent of self-doubt. When basic social science is so undeveloped compared with inquiry in the physical or life sciences, we might be asking ourselves, how could it be used to spawn an applied science that actually works? Obviously it cannot, and we ignore it.

Alternatively, the knowledge that there exists an effective science of political manipulation—if that is what it is—is discomfitting, and we choose to ignore it. It is hardly apt to compare the practice of strategic public diplomacy with the dropping of the first atomic bomb, but the issues raised for social scientists by the former phenomenon are in a sense not greatly different from those presented to physicists by the latter. My god, one might proclaim. The science works! What do we do now? It may more closely resemble Skinner's box than Pandora's, but the top is up.

Finally, and perhaps most plausibly, it may be that the institutions of science—the journals, graduate programs, professional associations, and the like—are always slow to recognize the value of new approaches. While we are scarcely talking here of paradigm-level change in the Kuhnian sense, the strain to preserve the conceptual status quo is a real one, and it is surely operating in this instance. And that is not altogether a bad thing. Not all new approaches are equally valid merely for having been propounded.

But whatever the reason for its present state, inquiry must now catch up with reality. And in the real world, strategic public diplomacy is a phenomenon of great scale, vigor, and effect.

Conclusion

I began this exercise with a caution that the research reported here is exploratory in nature. I have ended with at least a de facto assertion that it is definitive. Thus I have at once covered my behind—to adapt a term of some currency—and stuck out my neck. In combination, this is an uncomfortable position. And besides, the truth probably lies somewhere between the two extremes.

There is, I think, a good deal more significance to the subject of strategic public diplomacy than one might conclude from a review of the literature on U.S. foreign policy. The limited selection of content analyses and case studies I have been able to present here only begins to suggest the true dimensions of the phenomenon. Many, and more interesting, studies of individual campaigns and of class-level actions and effects await the researchers' examination. The work is basic to the development of the science of persuasion and to political science, and it is, at the same time, applied to a genuine problem that will be of growing societal importance. For both reasons, it is work worth pursuing. I hope these pages have intrigued and enlightened, but most of all I hope that they have encouraged the pursuit.

APPENDIX A

Selected Figures

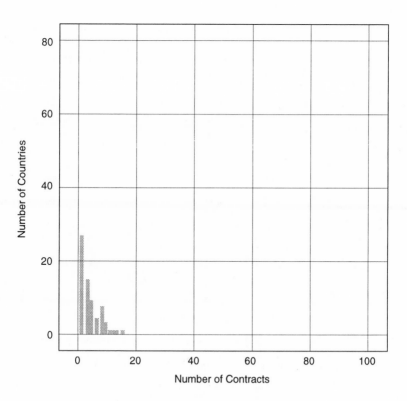

Figure A.1. Contracts for tourism services: 1987

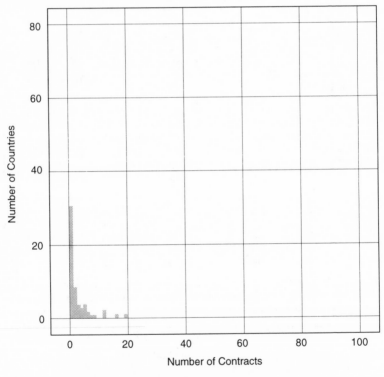

Figure A.2. Contracts for commercial services: 1987

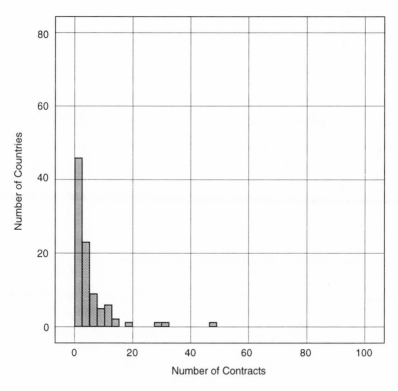

Figure A.3. Contracts for information services: 1987

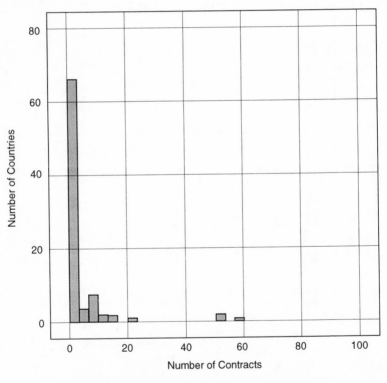

Figure A.4. Contracts for lobbying services: 1987

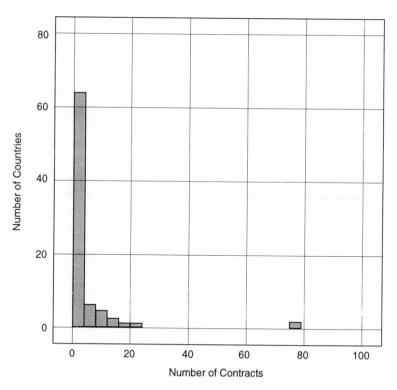

Figure A.5. Contracts for advice/research: 1987

APPENDIX B

Controlling for Regression
Toward the Mean

To address the possibility that the data reported in Figure 7.4 might be reflecting nothing more than regression toward the long-term mean values of news coverage, we selected three countries—Argentina, the Republic of Korea, and Turkey—for which we randomly selected for analysis two sets of twelve monthly time points, one for a three-year period and one for a ten-year period, each terminating in the date of the contract signing. We determined the mean values of each of our indicators for each of the months in question, then aggregated in three- and ten-year clusters to derive estimates of "normal" intermediate- and long-term coverage. The results of this analysis for two key variables— the number of insertions per month and the percentage of all valenced insertions that could be characterized as positive—are reported in Table B.1, published here for the first time.

If one regards three-year means as the more appropriate standard for assessing regression effects—and there is an argument to be made for doing so based in part on the pace of change in the international system and in part on the short memories of journalists and the public—then the data reported in Table B.1 suggest that, in every instance, the number of insertions, rather than regressing toward the mean, blasted well through it during the posttest period, ending up in two of the cases, Argentina and Korea, further from the mean in the opposite direction than was the point at which each started. And in all three instances, valence moved very substantially further from "normal" levels in the posttest than it had been in the pretest.

Using the ten-year standard of comparison, the results are a bit more

Appendices

mixed, but still somewhat supportive of an interpretation of substantive change. The weakest support comes from Argentina, where visibility moved directly to the ten-year mean, though valence moved through and slightly beyond that mark. The strongest support comes from Korea, where visibility moved well below long-term levels and valence moved strongly away from the mean. In the Turkish case, visibility trended toward the mean while valence moved sharply away.

Table B.1. Comparison of Preintervention and Postintervention Observations with Intermediate- and Long-Term Means

Country	Variable	Means			
		Pre	Post	3-Year	10-Year
Argentina	Inserts	21.6	10.9	16.9	10.7
	Valence	.10	.22	.11	.18
Korea	Inserts	18.3	7.6	15.9	12.8
	Valence	.23	.55	.20	.30
Turkey	Inserts	17.5	8.3	10.2	5.8
	Valence	.25	.60	.31	.32

APPENDIX C

List of Persons Interviewed

The analysis in this book is based in part on numerous conversations and interviews with scholars, journalists, public relations consultants, and officials of the United States and other governments that have taken place over more than a decade. A few of these have profoundly and directly shaped portions of the analysis. Those among them who have not requested anonymity are listed here by name (and by the position each held at the time of the interview) as an expression of my appreciation.

Allsop, Dee T., vice president for communications/marketing research, The Wirthlin Group.

Dayakar, Ratakonda, counsellor for public affairs, Embassy of India (Washington).

Fetig, James, lieutenant colonel, U.S. Army; special assistant for public affairs to the chief of staff of the Army; communication coordinator, Chief of Staff of the Army Assessments and Initiatives Group.

Fitz-Pegado, Lauri J., senior vice president and managing director, international public affairs division, Hill and Knowlton Public Affairs Worldwide.

Lee, Jong Ryool, chief press secretary and spokesman for the president of the Republic of Korea.

Mankiewicz, Frank, vice chairman and managing director, public affairs, Hill and Knowlton Public Affairs Worldwide.

Siegel, Mark A., president, Mark A. Siegel and Associates, Inc.; International Public Strategies, Inc.

Yoon, Ki Byung, secretary to the president (Republic of Korea) for political affairs.

In addition, several chapters incorporate research that I completed during three visits to the Republic of Korea during the period 1987 to 1989. Those visits were generously supported variously by the office of the press secretary to the president, the Korea Press Center, and the International Cultural Society of Korea. In the course of my visits, I had the opportunity to meet with a number of leaders of the Korean academy, media, and government. They are listed below by position held.

Minister of state for political affairs.

Minister, National Reunification Board.

Vice minister of culture and information.

Director, Korean Overseas Information Service.

Director general for foreign press, Korean Overseas Information Service.

Director, Press Relations Division, Korean Overseas Information Service.

Chairman, Foreign Affairs Committee, National Assembly (and other members of the National Assembly).

Press attache, Embassy of the Republic of Korea (Washington).

Member of the National Policy Coordination Committee and 1987 presidential campaign chairman, Democratic Justice party.

Secretary for foreign press relations, Reunification Democratic party.

Assistant dean for research, Institute of Foreign Affairs and National Security, Ministry of Foreign Affairs.

Managing editor, International Department, Yonhap News Agency.

Chairman, Korea Press Center.

Manager, press relations, Korea Press Center.

Deputy secretary general for international relations, Seoul Olympic Organizing Committee.

Director of academic affairs, Graduate School of the Academy of Korean Studies.

Executive director, International Cultural Society of Korea.

Director, Department of Cultural Affairs, International Cultural Society of Korea.

General Manager, Trade Cooperation Department, Korea Foreign Trade Association.

Scholars in the fields of international relations, political science, mass communication, journalism, and sociology at Seoul National University, Yonsei University, Korea University, Sogang University, and Myung Gi University.

Senior journalists with two Korean newspapers.

President, Seoul Foreign Correspondents' Club, and other Western journalists covering Korean affairs.

And in Washington, the desk officer for Korean affairs of the U.S. Department of State.

My thanks as well to everyone else who contributed so generously of their time and expertise to help educate me as to the ways of public diplomacy.

Notes

Chapter 1

1. For examples of this work, see Hovland, Lumsdaine, and Sheffield, 1949; and Institute of Communications Research, 1955.

2. Actually, for a brief period at the time of the report this agency was called the International Communication Agency, a name soon discarded because of the similarity of its acronym with that of the CIA.

3. Though working within this general framework, Signitzer and Coombs (1991) do take a more conceptual approach, arguing for a more explicit convergence of public relations practice with theories of cultural communication.

4. For a recent compendium of research findings regarding persuasion, many of which underlie the theory and practice of strategic communication, see O'Keefe, 1990. This perspective also draws on applications of persuasion theory developed in the field of issues management, which focuses on corporate image making and the importance to corporate interests of public opinion. For an overview of developments in this field, see Heath and Nelson, 1986. Finally, for an analysis that applies the techniques of new-product marketing to the management of political images, see Mauser, 1983.

5. Interestingly enough, and directly on point, the endowment became a political football during the congressional budget debate of 1993, when it was zeroed out of the House of Representatives' version of the federal budget, an indication of the low priority assigned to its activities by many in the Congress.

Chapter 2

1. The analysis reported here is subject to several limitations. First, though registration requirements were first instituted in 1938, organized reporting of the results was not begun until 1950, when a report covering the period 1947–50 was issued. The first of the attorney general's annual reports was issued the following year. For reasons stated below, the present analysis actually begins with the report for 1967. Second, because of changing requirements, both legislative and political, the form of the attorney general's report has changed from time to time, with particular data being included or excluded at various points in the series. This results in some missing data problems, though generally the more recent reports are the most complete. Third, the collection of reports in the Department of Justice library is incomplete. As a result, the present research excludes data for the years 1972 and 1974. Fourth, and perhaps most significantly, there is some question regarding the level of compliance with the reporting requirements under FARA. One concern, in particular, is language employed in the act that defines virtually any activities related to the development and dissemination of political information as "propaganda." At least one member of Congress, Dan Glickman (D-KS), believes this language is sufficiently pejorative to discourage contractors from filing reports or from characterizing their activities appropriately. He has introduced a series of proposed FARA amendments that would have the effect, among others, of changing the description of these activities. As Glickman (1991) himself stated on the House floor,

> . . . My legislation attempts to get rid of the stigma attached to the label "foreign agent," which is commonly believed to cause great reluctance to register with the Justice Department. It is widely held that the approximately 900 persons currently registered represent only a fraction of the total who should register under FARA. FARA would be renamed as the "Foreign Interests Representation Act." The term "political propaganda" would also be dropped in favor of "promotional or informational materials." Other negative terms like "indoctrinate" and "convert" would be replaced by the neutral term "influence."

Another aspect of compliance relates to the financial reporting requirements under the act. The extensive review of 1987 registrations to be reported below, for example, identified 250 instances in which services were performed, but for which no remuneration was reported. This is a relatively small proportion of total contracts, and not all of these cases represent noncompliance. Some are the product of multiple-client contracts where one client paid the full costs. Others represent filings of intended future services, while still more are attributable to voluntary efforts or the activities of cause groups. A small number (I estimate perhaps 10 percent based on a review of the reverse circumstance in which fees are collected but no services are provided during the reporting period) result from a time lag between the provision of services and the receipt of compensation. And still others may actually be the foreign agent equivalent of loss leaders, the provision of complementary services in anticipation that they will lead to revenue-generating contracts at a later date. Nevertheless, it seems likely that some 40 to 50 percent of these cases may represent some form of noncompliance.

Finally, it is important to note inherent limitations of some of the coding categories reported below. Although I have made an effort to categorize the data in the attorney general's reports carefully and systematically, this is inevitably a highly judgmental process. The language in each record is that of the registrant, and many of the registrants are professional wordsmiths concerned, as Representative Glickman suggests, about their own images as well as the interests of their clients. Thus, one must engage in some measure of interpretation in developing an understanding of what was involved in each contract. Similarly, financial reports have been aggregated (in the most recent reports) at the contract level, but a single contract may be the basis for providing several diverse services. This, too, requires interpretation. These and other factors pose potential threats to the reliability of the data. Resources did not permit the employment of multiple coders or the assessment of intercoder reliability for this portion of the research. Based on past experience, I cannot say with confidence that reliability measures for some of the indicators reported here would have achieved the 90 percent reliability generally required in such undertakings.

2. Not all consulting firms have chosen to enter the international arena, at least as representatives of governmental interests. At least one of the most prominent Washington public relations firms, for example, eschews such clients. The partners in the firm put the question to their staff, who decided against taking on such clients, in no small measure because of the potential liabilities to the firm's image of being associated in the public mind with a coterie of LDCs— Lesser Desired Clients.

3. These data are not affected by the anomaly that led to the exclusion of 1987 from the summary reported in Table 2.1.

4. This included, for example, activity other than tourism contracted directly by a foreign government, activity directly related to any function of the U.S. government or to U.S. public policy, or activity expressly defined in the registration statement as political in character.

5. FARA reports include as "countries" such entities as South Moluccas, Palestine, Puerto Rico, and a category labeled "International," which includes both multinational contracts and those undertaken by international organizations such as the European Community.

6. These data are derived from appendices in the attorney general's report for that year and are at some variance with aggregates based on analysis of the raw data, but probably not in ways material to the present analysis.

7. We already know, of course, that many of the largest contracts are assigned to the less populous of these categories. Ideally, then, we should review a similar set of figures based on expenditures related to each activity and on that basis further enlighten our understanding of the relative weights of each service class in the overall industry. Unfortunately, the data are not reported by the Justice Department—and are probably not made available to the department—in a manner that is conducive to such an analysis.

Chapter 3

1. Fitz-Pegado left Hill and Knowlton in 1993 to accept a position with the Department of Commerce.
2. After a public outcry, Ms. Daponte was reinstated.

Chapter 5

1. Table 5.3 below includes data on the thematic content of *Post* coverage of Pakistan, which does not show any increased attention to the theme of "democracy" following Bhutto's visit. This may be misleading because the "political affairs" heading in the newspaper's indexing system—which was used as a criterion for organizing the analysis reported in the table—does not generally include coverage of a country's foreign affairs activities, and there was, in fact, some coverage of the democracy theme in the newspaper's reporting on the visit itself. Still, if there was a payoff in the *Post,* it was not an immediate one.
2. The inclusion of these items was not entirely systematic, but there is no reason to suspect any nonrandom variation in selection during the period surrounding the Bhutto visit. Thus while analysis based on transcripts in the database is not inclusive, any existing bias in the selection process is not likely to be related to, or affect, the subject of the present study.
3. Murray Edelman, in *The Symbolic Uses of Politics;* Charles Elder and Roger Cobb, in *The Political Uses of Symbols;* and others have long suggested the importance of language choice in politics. The correct word or symbol can be applied to frame issues and establish constituencies for particular points of view; to set standards of judgment; to frighten, reassure, unify, or divide populations; and to a host of other purposes.

Among the key elements of the image of any attitude object are the verbal or other cues with which that object is regularly associated either in media portrayals or in the public mind. Elder and Cobb (1983: 35–56) argue that these cues can be either substantive or associational in character—focusing in the first instance on perceived attributes of the primary attitude object itself and in the second on perceived attributes of the social context in which the object is presented.

Combs (1980), Bennett (1988a), and others have pointed out the tendency of news organizations and the public affairs media generally to emphasize the dramatic aspects of politics in their portrayals of persons and events. Bennett, in particular, argues that story lines develop that are used as a shorthand device for conveying a sense of context—as distinct from its substance—to the audience. To this end, specific cues are employed to establish the continuity of long-running stories. At the other end of the pipeline, Graber (1988) shows how members of the news audience draw on existing schema—frameworks of understanding—to assign meaning to the news they receive. Both arguments are dependent in some measure on the presence in the news of thematic cues. Indeed, Entman (1991) suggests that such cues are an inherent component of the news itself.

4. Hartwig (1990) argues that American responsiveness to such appeals actually represents a significant point of vulnerability in U.S. foreign policy and, in his view, one not worth the risk.

5. The selection of target countries for this analysis was entirely judgmental. The objective was to identify five countries from each of four areas of the world, each of which had been the locus of actual or prospective fundamental political change—where possible, involving forces that might in some way be described as democratic—during the period of analysis. Each region contained a mix of major and minor countries (with respect to their apparent newsworthiness), and the regions themselves varied in the amount of attention they were accorded in the newspaper.

6. This number is inflated by double coding—articles that mentioned more than one of the target countries—but for purposes of the present research each country-insertion has been treated as a separate item.

Chapter 6

1. For an analysis of the latter point as it applied to the Persian Gulf War, see Hallin and Gitlin (1993).

2. Data reported here are drawn from the *Statistical Abstract of the United States* (1987) and from reports produced by the Korean government.

3. Even today, though both sides have moved toward a raprochement, officials express distrust of North Korean motives and sincerity with respect to reunification.

4. Shoemaker, Danielian, and Brendlinger (1988) show that *Times* coverage of foreign affairs is allocated according to the apparent political importance of

the subject country. Bennett (1990) suggests that the relationship between media and the policy elite, at least with respect to the *Times*, is circular, with the newspaper taking its cues from the same elite audience whose views it then helps to shape.

5. No effort has been made here to segregate counts of economic and political news *within* each newspaper. To the extent that political news drives the coverage in the *Journal* or economic news that in the *Times*, any relationship cited between the two types of coverage is likely to be overstated.

6. An interesting and perhaps ironic sidebar to the 1964 games is that they were the first in which a team from North Korea was permitted to participate.

7. Because of its derivation, the correlation coefficient is interpreted such that the square of its value represents the proportion of variance in a dependent variable attributable to the influence on it of the independent variable.

Chapter 7

1. For a detailed examination of inoculation strategies as they are applied in domestic politics, see Pfau and Kenski (1990). The logic of the strategy is essentially the same when it is applied in foreign affairs.

2. In terms of the agenda dynamics model to be developed in Chapter 8, this would be described as embedding the image in salience cues.

3. As some readers will note after completing Chapter 8, some of these indicators (e.g., reliability) relate to salience cues that were not analytically distinguished from valence at the time this research was conducted.

4. We regarded this as a more rigorous test of our formulation than would have been the random selection of countries and time points that some critics at the time suggested.

5. The firm later denied that it had undertaken any "political" work for Iran and resigned from the account.

Chapter 9

1. Mauser (1983: 5) has termed it a "managerial" technology.

Bibliography

Abshire, David M. (1976). *International Broadcasting: A New Dimension of Western Diplomacy*. Beverly Hills, CA: Sage.

Adams, William C. (1987). "Mass Media and Public Opinion About Foreign Affairs: A Typology of News Dynamics," *Political Communication and Persuasion* 4: 263–78.

Albritton, Robert B., and Jarol B. Manheim (1983). "News of Rhodesia: The Impact of a Public Relations Campaign," *Journalism Quarterly* 60: 622–28.

——— (1985). "Public Relations Efforts for the Third World: Images in the News," *Journal of Communication* 35: 43–59.

Amaize, Odekhiren, and Ronald J. Faber (1983). "Advertising by National Governments in Leading United States, Indian and British Newspapers," *Gazette* 32: 87–101.

Andersen, Robin (1989). "The Reagan Administration and Nicaragua: The Use of Public Diplomacy to Influence Media Coverage and Public Opinion," paper presented at the annual meeting of the Speech Communication Association, San Francisco.

Anonymous (1991a). "Nine firms working for Kuwait; big $ to Rendon, Neill, CGS&H," *O'Dwyer's FARA Report* 1 (March). New York: J. R. O'Dwyer, pp. 1–2.

——— (1991b). "Hill and Knowlton's six-month FARA fees hit $14.2 million," *O'Dwyer's FARA Report* 1 (July). New York: J. R. O'Dwyer, pp. 1–2.

——— (1991c). "Kuwait awards PR to Keene, Shirley," *O'Dwyer's FARA Report* 1 (July): 1. New York: J. R. O'Dwyer.

——— (1991d). "Citizens for Free Kuwait files with FARA after nine-month lag," *O'Dwyer's FARA Report* I: 9 (October). New York: J. R. O'Dwyer, pp. 1-2.

Attorney General of the United States (1987 and others). *Report of the Attorney General to the Congress of the United States on the Administration of the Foreign Agents Registration Act of 1938, as Amended, for the Calendar Year. . . .* Washington: U.S. Department of Justice.

Auerbach, Stuart (1991). "Kuwaitis Paid for Mosbacher Trip," *Washington Post,* June 5: A13.

Becker, Lee B. (1977). "Foreign Policy and Press Performance," *Journalism Quarterly* 54: 364–68.

Behr, R. L., and Shanto Iyengar (1985). "Television News, Real World Cues, and Changes in the Public Agenda," *Public Opinion Quarterly* 49: 38–57.

Bender, M. (1976). "Marion Javits Issue Focuses Unwelcome Spotlight on Publicizing of Foreign Clients," *New York Times,* February 27: 6.

Bennett, W. Lance (1988a). *News: The Politics of Illusion,* 2d ed. White Plains, NY: Longman.

———— (1988b). "Marginalizing the Majority: The News Media, Public Opinion, and Nicaragua Policy Decisions," in Michael Margolis and Gary Mauser, eds., *Manipulating Public Opinion.* Pacific Grove, CA: Brooks/Cole, pp. 320–61.

———— (1990). "Toward a Theory of Press-State Relations in the United States," *Journal of Communication* 40: 103–25.

Bennett, W. Lance, and Jarol B. Manheim (1993). "Taking the Public by Storm: Information, Cuing, and the Democratic Process in the Gulf Conflict," *Political Communication* 10: 331–52.

Benton, M., and P. J. Frazier (1976). "The Agenda-Setting Function of Mass Media at Three Levels of 'Information Holding,'" *Communication Research* 3: 261–74.

Berkowitz, D. (1987). "Television News Sources and News Channels: A Study in Agenda Building," *Journalism Quarterly* 64: 508–13.

Bolce, Louis, Gerald DeMaio, and Douglas Muzzio (1987). "The Equal Rights Amendment, Public Opinion, and American Constitutionalism," *Polity* 19: 551–69.

Booker, Christopher (1981). *The Games War: A Moscow Journal.* London: Faber and Faber.

Brody, Richard A. (1991). "Crisis, War, and Public Opinion: The Media and Public Support for the President in Two Phases of the Confrontation in the Persian Gulf, Part I," paper presented at the Social Science Research Council Conference on Media and Foreign Policy, Seattle.

Brosius, Hans-Bernd, and Hans Mathias Kepplinger (1990). "Linear and Nonlinear Models of Agenda Setting in Television," paper presented at the annual meeting of the International Communication Association, Dublin, Ireland.

Cambridge, Vibert C. (1988). "'Project Democracy' and U.S. Public Diplomacy," paper presented at the annual meeting of the International Communication Association, New Orleans.

Center for Public Integrity (1993). *The Trading Game: Inside Lobbying for the North American Free Trade Agreement.* Washington, DC.

Charles, Jeff, Larry Shore, and Rusty Todd (1979). "The *New York Times* Coverage of Equatorial and Lower Africa," *Journal of Communication* 29: 148–55.

Choate, Pat (1990). *Agents of Influence.* New York: Alfred A. Knopf.

Cobb, Roger W., and Charles D. Elder (1972). *Participation in American Politics: The Dynamics of Agenda Building.* Boston: Allyn & Bacon.

Cobb, Roger W., Jenny Ross, and M. H. Ross (1976). "Agenda Building as a Comparative Political Process," *American Political Science Review* 70: 126–38.

Cohen, Bernard (1963). *The Press and Foreign Policy.* Princeton, NJ: Princeton University Press.

——— (1973). *The Public's Impact on Foreign Policy.* Boston: Little, Brown.

Cohen, Raymond (1987). *Theatre of Power: The Art of Diplomatic Signalling.* London: Longman.

Cohen, Yoel (1988). "Military Information, the News Media, and the Falklands Conflict," in *Israel Yearbook on Human Rights,* Vol. 18. Tel Aviv: Faculty of Law, Tel Aviv University, pp. 87–100.

Combs, James E. (1980). *Dimensions of Political Drama.* Santa Monica, CA: Goodyear.

Cook, F. L., and D. S. King (1982). "Toward a Theory of Issue Decline on Policy Agendas," paper presented at the Symposium on New Directions in the Empirical and Normative Study of Public Policy, Northwestern University, Evanston, IL.

Curtis, Bill (1983). *On Assignment with Bill Curtis.* Chicago: Rand McNally, p. 134. Also in an interview on *Morning Edition,* National Public Radio, December 13.

Cushman, John H., Jr. (1992). "U.S. Offers Proof of Iraqi Atrocity," *New York Times,* February 6: A11.

Czudnowski, Morris M. (1968). "A Salience Dimension of Politics for the Study of Political Culture," *American Political Science Review* 62: 878–88.

Davis, Morris (1977). *Interpreters for Nigeria: The Third World and International Public Relations.* Urbana: University of Illinois Press.

Davison, W. Philips (1974). "News Media and International Negotiation," *Public Opinion Quarterly* 38: 174–93.

Deaver, Michael K. (1987). *Behind the Scenes.* New York: William Morrow and Company.

Deibel, Terry L., and Walter R. Roberts (1976). *Culture and Information: Two Foreign Policy Functions*. The Washington Papers, Vol. IV, no. 40. Beverly Hills, CA: Sage.

DeParle, Jason (1991). "Long Series of Military Decisions Led to Gulf War News Censorship," *New York Times,* May 5: A1, A20.

Dorman, William A., and Steven Livingston (1992). "Historical Content and the News: Policy Consequences for the 1990–91 Persian Gulf Crisis," paper presented at the annual meeting of the International Communication Association, Miami.

Downs, Anthony (1972). "Up and Down with Ecology: The 'Issue-Attention Cycle,'" *The Public Interest* 28: 38–50.

Edelman, Murray (1964). *The Symbolic Uses of Politics*. Urbana: University of Illinois Press.

———— (1971). *Politics as Symbolic Action: Mass Arousal and Quiescence*. Chicago: Markham.

———— (1988). *Constructing the Political Spectacle*. Chicago: University of Chicago Press.

Einseidel, E. F., K. L. Salomone, and F. P. Schneider (1984). "Crime: Effects of Media Exposure and Personal Experience on Issue Salience," *Journalism Quarterly* 61: 131–36.

Elder, Charles D., and Roger W. Cobb (1983). *The Political Uses of Symbols*. New York: Longman.

Entman, Robert M. (1991). "Framing U.S. Coverage of International News: Contrasts in Narratives of the KAL and Iran Air Incidents," *Journal of Communication* 41: 6–27.

Erbring, Lutz, Edie N. Goldenberg, and Arthur Miller (1980). "Front-Page News and Real-World Cues: A New Look at Agenda-Setting by the Media," *American Journal of Political Science* 24: 16–49.

Erfle, Stephen, Henry McMillan, and Bernard Grofman (1990). "Regulation via Threats: Politics, Media Coverage, and Oil Pricing Decisions," *Public Opinion Quarterly* 54: 48–63.

Espy, Richard (1979). *The Politics of the Olympic Games*. Berkeley: University of California Press.

Eyal, Chaim (1980). *Time Frame in Agenda-Setting Research: A Study of the Conceptual and Methodological Factors Affecting the Time-Frame Context of the Agenda-Setting Process*. Unpublished doctoral dissertation, Syracuse University, as cited in Maxwell E. McCombs, "The Agenda-Setting Approach," in Dan D. Nimmo and Keith R. Saunders, eds., *Handbook of Political Communication*. Beverly Hills, CA: Sage, 1981.

Festinger, Leon (1957). *A Theory of Cognitive Dissonance*. Evanston, IL: Row, Peterson.

Fisher, Glen H. (1972). *Public Diplomacy and the Behavioral Sciences.* Bloomington: Indiana University Press.

———— (1987). *American Communication in a Global Society,* rev. ed. Norwood, NJ: Ablex.

Gantz, W., S. Trenholm, and M. Pitman (1976). "The Impact of Salience and Altruism on Diffusion of News," *Journalism Quarterly* 53: 727–32.

Gellman, Barton (1992). "Census Worker Who Calculated '91 Iraqi Death Toll Is Told She Will Be Fired," *Washington Post,* March 6: A6.

Gitlin, Todd (1991). Commentary at the Social Science Research Council Conference on Media and Foreign Policy, Seattle.

Glickman, Dan (1991). *Congressional Record,* April 11: H2169.

Graber, Doris A. (1988). *Processing the News: How People Tame the Information Tide,* 2d ed. New York: Longman.

Grau, C. H. (1976). "What Publications Are Most Frequently Quoted in the *Congressional Record?*" *Journalism Quarterly* 53: 716–19.

Green, Donald P., and Ann E. Gerken (1989). "Self Interest and Opinion Toward Smoking Restrictions and Cigarette Taxes," *Public Opinion Quarterly* 53: 1–16.

Green, Fitzhugh (1988). *American Propaganda Abroad: From Benjamin Franklin to Ronald Reagan.* New York: Hippocrene Books.

Green, John C., and James L. Guth (1989). "The Missing Link: Political Activists and Support for School Prayer," *Public Opinion Quarterly* 53: 41–57.

Greenberg, A., and N. Garfinkle (1963). "Visual Material and Recall of Magazine Articles," *Journal of Advertising Research* 3: 30–34.

Hallin, Daniel C., and Todd Gitlin (1993). "Agon and Ritual: The Gulf War as Popular Culture and as Television Drama," *Political Communication* 10: 411–24.

Harrington, David E. (1989). "Economic News on Television: The Determinants of Coverage," *Public Opinion Quarterly* 53: 17–40.

Hart, D. V. (1977). "The Filipino-American Press in the United States: A Neglected Resource," *Journalism Quarterly* 54: 135–39.

Hart-Davis, Duff (1986). *Hitler's Games: The 1936 Olympics.* London: Century Hutchinson Ltd.

Hartwig, Richard (1990). "Democracy as an Objective of United States Foreign Policy," paper presented at the annual meeting of the Midwest Political Science Association, Chicago.

Hazan, Baruch (1982). *Olympic Sports and Propaganda Games: Moscow 1980.* New Brunswick, NJ: Transaction.

Heath, Robert L., and Richard A. Nelson (1986). *Issues Management: Corporate Public Policymaking in an Information Society.* Beverly Hills, CA: Sage.

Hiatt, Fred, and Margaret Shapiro (1988). "Wealthy Japan Devises a New Role as Aid Donor and World Power," *Washington Post*, June 3: A21, A28.

Hill and Knowlton (1967, 1968). *Handbook on International Public Relations*, Vols. 1 and 2. New York: Praeger.

——— (1990). "Facts and History," unpublished corporate materials.

——— (n.d.). "International Public Affairs: The Power of Communication," unpublished corporate materials.

Hoberman, John M. (1984). *Sport and Political Ideology*. Austin: University of Texas Press.

——— (1986). *The Olympic Crisis: Sport, Politics and the Moral Order*. New Rochelle, NY: Caratzas Publishing.

Hoffman, Arthur S., ed. (1968). *International Communication and the New Diplomacy*. Bloomington: Indiana University Press.

Hopple, Gerald W. (1982). "International News Coverage in Two Elite Newspapers," *Journal of Communication* 32: 61–74.

Hovland, Carl I., Arthur A. Lumsdaine, and Fred D. Sheffield (1949). *Experiments on Mass Communication*, Vol. 3. New York: John Wiley & Sons.

Howe, Russell W., and Sarah H. Trott (1976). *The Power Peddlers: How Lobbyists Mold America's Foreign Policy*. Garden City, NY: Doubleday, 1977.

Hvistendahl, J. K. (1968). "The Effect of Subheads on Reader Comprehension," *Journalism Quarterly* 45: 123–25.

Institute of Communications Research (1955). *Four Working Papers on Propaganda Theory*. Urbana: University of Illinois.

International Cultural Society of Korea (1986 and others). *ICSK: Annual Report*. Seoul, Korea: ICSK serial.

Iyengar, Shanto (1990). "Framing Responsibility for Political Issues: The Case of Poverty," *Political Behavior* 12: 19–40.

Javits, Jacob K. (1981). *Javits: The Autobiography of a Public Man*. Boston: Houghton Mifflin.

Jennings, M. Kent, and L. Harmon Zeigler (1970). "The Salience of State Politics Among Attentive Publics," in Edward C. Dreyer and Walter C. Rosenbaum, eds., *Political Opinion and Behavior*, 2d ed. Belmont, CA: Wadsworth.

Kent, K. E., and R. R. Rush (1976). "How Communication Behavior of Older Persons Affects Their Public Affairs Knowledge," *Journalism Quarterly* 53: 40–46.

Kingdon, John (1984). *Agendas, Alternatives, and Public Policies*. Boston: Little, Brown.

Kotler, Phillip (1982). *Marketing for Nonprofit Organizations*, 2d ed. Englewood Cliffs, NJ: Prentice-Hall.

Krauss, Clifford (1992). "Congressman Says Girl Was Credible," *New York Times* (January 12): A11.

Kriesel, Melvin E. (1985). "Psychological Operations: A Strategic View," in *Essays on Strategy: Selections from the 1984 Joint Chiefs of Staff Essay Competition*. Washington: National Defense University Press.

Krosnick, Jon A. (1990). "Government Policy and Citizen Passion: A Study of Issue Publics in Contemporary America," *Political Behavior* 12: 59–92.

Krugman, Herbert E. (1965). "The Impact of Television Advertising: Learning Without Involvement," *Public Opinion Quarterly* 29: 349–56.

Lachica, E. (1982). "Philippines Makes Lavish Preparations for President Marcos's State Visit to U.S.," *Wall Street Journal*, September 14: 36.

Lane, Robert E., and David O. Sears (1964). *Public Opinion*. Englewood Cliffs, NJ: Prentice-Hall.

Lang, Gladys E., and Kurt Lang (1981). "Watergate: An Exploration of the Agenda Building Process," in G. G. Wilhoit and H. deBock, eds., *Mass Communication Review Yearbook*, Vol. 2. Beverly Hills, CA: Sage, pp. 447–68.

Larson, James F. (1989). "'Seoul to the World': The Televised Olympic Spectacle and Intercultural Understanding," paper presented at the Seoul Olympiad Anniversary Conference, Seoul, South Korea.

Lee, Alfred M. (1952). *How to Understand Propaganda*. New York: Rinehart & Company.

Lee, John, ed. (1968). *The Diplomatic Persuaders: New Role of the Mass Media in International Relations*. New York: John Wiley & Sons.

Leff, Donna R., David L. Protess, and Stephen C. Brooks (1986). "Crusading Journalism: Changing Public Attitudes and Policy-Making Agendas," *Public Opinion Quarterly* 50: 300–15.

Lent, John A. (1977). "Foreign News in American Media," *Journal of Communication* 27: 46–51.

Maass, Peter (1988). "NBC's Olympic Trials," *Washington Post*, July 7: C1, C10–11.

MacArthur, John R. (1992). *Second Front: Censorship and Propaganda in the Gulf War*. New York: Hill and Wang.

Malone, Gifford D. (1988). *Political Advocacy and Cultural Communication: Organizing the Nation's Public Diplomacy*. Lanham, MD: University Press of America.

Mandell, Richard D. (1987). *The Nazi Olympics*. Urbana: University of Illinois Press.

Manheim, Jarol B. (1987). "A Model of Agenda Dynamics," in Margaret L. McLaughlin, ed., *Communication Yearbook 10*. Beverly Hills, CA: Sage, pp. 499–516.

—— (1988a). "Cultures in Conflict: External Communications and U.S.-Korean Relations," paper presented at the annual meeting of the International Communication Association, New Orleans.

—— (1988b). "Political Culture and Political Communication: Implications for U.S.-Korean Relations," paper presented at the annual meeting of the American Political Science Association, Washington, DC.

—— (1990a). "Rites of Passage: The 1988 Seoul Olympics as Public Diplomacy," *Western Political Quarterly:* 279–95.

—— (1990b). "Coming to America: Head-of-State Visits as Public Diplomacy," paper presented at the annual meeting of the International Communication Association, Dublin, Ireland.

—— (1990c). "'Democracy' as International Public Relations," paper presented at the annual meeting of the American Political Science Association, San Francisco.

—— (1991a). *All of the People, All the Time: Strategic Communication and American Politics.* Armonk, NY: M. E. Sharpe.

—— (1991b). "Image Making as an Instrument of Power: The Representation of Foreign Interests in the United States," paper presented at the annual meeting of the International Communication Association, Chicago.

—— (1991c). "All for a Good Cause: Managing Kuwait's Image During the Gulf Conflict," paper presented at the Social Science Research Council Conference on Media and Foreign Policy, Seattle.

—— (1991d). "Communication as a Weapon of War," paper presented at the Political Psychology of the Gulf War Conference, Graduate Center of the City University of New York, New York.

Manheim, Jarol B., and Robert B. Albritton (1984). "Changing National Images: International Public Relations and Media Agenda Setting," *American Political Science Review* 78: 641–54.

—— (1986). "Public Relations in the Public Eye: Two Case Studies of the Failure of Public Information Campaigns," *Political Communication and Persuasion* 3: 265–91.

—— (1987). "Insurgent Violence Versus Image Management: The Struggle for National Images in Southern Africa," *British Journal of Political Science* 17: 201–18.

Margolis, Michael, and Gary A. Mauser (1989). "Public Opinion as a Dependent Variable: A Framework for Analysis," *Political Communication and Persuasion* 6: 87–108.

Matlack, Carol (1991). "Dead in the Water?" *National Journal,* May 18: 1156–60.

Mauser, Gary A. (1983). *Political Marketing: An Approach to Campaign Strategy.* New York: Praeger.

McCombs, Maxwell E., and Donald L. Shaw (1972). "The Agenda-Setting Function of Mass Media," *Public Opinion Quarterly* 36: 176–87.

McGuire, William J. (1964). "Inducing Resistance to Persuasion: Some Contemporary Approaches," in L. Berkowitz, ed., *Advances in Experimental Social Psychology,* Vol. 1. New York: Academic Press, pp. 191–229.

Mehling, R. (1959). "Attitude Changing Effect of News and Photo Combinations," *Journalism Quarterly* 36: 189–98.

Merritt, Richard L. (1980). "Transforming International Communications Strategies," *Political Communication and Persuasion* 1: 5–42.

Modigliani, Andre, and Franco Modigliani (1987). "The Growth of the Federal Deficit and the Role of Public Attitudes," *Public Opinion Quarterly* 51: 459–80.

Molotch, H., and M. Lester (1974). "News as Purposive Behavior: On the Strategic Use of Routine Events, Accidents, and Scandals," *American Sociological Review* 39: 101–12.

Mueller, John (1988). "Trends in Political Tolerance," *Public Opinion Quarterly* 52: 1–25.

Mueller, Keith (1988). "The Role of Policy Analysis in Agenda Setting: Applications to the Problem of Indigent Health Care in the United States," *Policy Studies Journal* 16: 441–53.

Mufson, Steven (1992). "The Privatization of Craig Fuller," *Washington Post Magazine,* August 2: 14–19, 26–31.

National Public Radio (1982). "All Things Considered," September 14.

Nimmo, Dan, and James E. Combs (1983). *Mediated Political Realities.* New York: Longman.

O'Keefe, Daniel J. (1990). *Persuasion: Theory and Research.* Newbury Park, CA: Sage.

Page, Benjamin I., and Robert Y. Shapiro (1983). "Effects of Public Opinion on Policy," *American Political Science Review* 77: 175–90.

Page, Benjamin I., Robert Y. Shapiro, and Glenn R. Dempsey (1985). "The Mass Media Do Affect Policy Preferences," paper presented at the annual meeting of the American Association for Public Opinion Research, McAfee, NJ.

———— (1987). "What Moves Public Opinion?" *American Political Science Review* 81: 23–43.

Peterson, S. (1981). "International News Selection by the Elite Press," *Public Opinion Quarterly* 45: 143–63.

Pfau, Michael, and Henry Kenski (1990). *Attack Politics: Strategy and Defense.* New York: Praeger.

Powers, R. D., and B. E. Kearl (1968). "Readability and Display as Readership Predictors," *Journalism Quarterly* 45: 117–18.

Priest, Dana (1992a). "Kuwait Baby-Killing Report Disputed," *Washington Post,* February 7: A17.

—— (1992b). "Report Faults Iraqis in Babies' Death," *Washington Post,* June 30: A 14.

Pritchard, David (1986). "Homicide and Bargained Justice: The Agenda-Setting Effect of Crime News on Prosecutors," *Public Opinion Quarterly* 50: 143–59.

Radcliffe, Donnie (1982). "Marcos Plans Trip," *Washington Post,* August 10: C1, C8.

Radcliffe, Donnie, and Martha Sherrill (1989). "Bhutto, Back at the White House," *Washington Post,* June 7: C1, C8.

Rosellini, L. (1982). "The Panoply of Preparation for the Marcos Visit," *New York Times,* September 15, B8.

Rowland, Robert C., and Roger A. Payne (1987). "The Effectiveness of Reagan's 'Star Wars' Address," *Political Communication and Persuasion* 4: 161–78.

Salwen, Michael B. (1988). "Effect of Accumulation of Coverage on Issue Salience in Agenda Setting," *Journalism Quarterly* 65: 100–106.

Salwen, Michael B., and Bruce Garrison (1988). "What is Newsworthy and What is Not? A Comparison of U.S. and Latin American Gatekeepers," paper presented at the annual meeting of the International Communication Association, New Orleans.

Saunders, Harold (1988). " 'Us and Them'–Building Mature International Relationships: The Role of Official and Supplemental Diplomacy," presentation before the University Seminar in Political Psychology, George Washington University, Washington, DC, April 11.

Semmel, Andrew K. (1976). "Foreign News in Four U.S. Elite Dailies: Some Comparisons," *Journalism Quarterly* 53: 732–36.

Sharkey, Jacqueline (1991). *Under Fire: U.S. Military Restrictions on the Media from Grenada to the Persian Gulf.* Washington, DC.: Center for Public Integrity.

Shaw, Donald (1992). Personal conversation.

Shaw, Donald L., and Maxwell E. McCombs (1977). *The Emergence of American Political Issues: The Agenda-Setting Function of the Press.* St. Paul, MN: West.

Shoemaker, Pamela J., Lucig H. Danielian, and Nancy Brendlinger (1988). "Deviant Acts, Risky Business, and U.S. Interests: The Newsworthiness of World Events," paper presented at the annual meeting of the International Communication Association, New Orleans.

Sigal, Leon V. (1973). *Reporters and Officials: The Organization and Politics of Newsmaking.* Lexington, MA: D. C. Heath.

Sigelman, Lee, James Lebovic, Clyde Wilcox, and Dee Allsop (1993). "As Time Goes By: Daily Opinion Change During the Persian Gulf Crisis," *Political Communication* 10: 353–68.

Signitzer, Benno, and Timothy Coombs (1991). "Public Relations and Public Diplomacy: Conceptual Convergences," *Public Relations Review* 17: 137–47.

Smith, Anthony (1980). *The Geopolitics of Information: How Western Culture Dominates the World*. New York: Oxford University Press.

Smith, Hedrick (1988). *The Power Game*. New York: Random House.

Strong, Morgan (1992). "Portions of the Gulf War were brought to you by the folks at Hill and Knowlton," *TV Guide*, February 22: 11–13.

Taylor, Trevor (1986). "Politics and the Olympic Spirit," in Lincoln Allison, ed., *The Politics of Sport*. Manchester, England: University of Manchester Press, pp. 216–41.

Tuch, Hans N. (1990). *Communicating with the World: U.S. Public Diplomacy Overseas*. New York: St. Martin's Press.

Tyler, Patrick E. (1988). "Kurds Disappoint Iraqi PR Effort," *Washington Post*, September 18: A30.

United States Department of Commerce (1987). *Statistical Abstract of the United States 1987*. Washington, DC: U.S. Government Printing Office.

United States General Accounting Office (1979). *The Public Diplomacy of Other Countries: Implications for the United States*. Washington, DC: Government Printing Office.

——— (1992). *Foreign Agent Registration: Former Federal Officials Representing Foreign Interests Before the U.S. Government*. Washington, DC: Government Printing Office.

United States House of Representatives (1977). *Public Diplomacy and the Future*. Hearings before the Subcommittee on International Operations of the Committee on International Relations. Washington, DC: U.S.G.P.O.

——— (1987). *Oversight of Public Diplomacy*. Hearings before the Subcommittee on International Operations of the Committee on Foreign Affairs. Washington, DC: U.S.G.P.O.

Verba, Sidney, and Norman H. Nie (1972). *Participation in America: Political Democracy and Social Equality*. New York: Harper & Row.

Wayne, Stephen (1993). "President Bush Goes to War: A Psychological Interpretation from a Distance," in Stanley A. Renshon, ed., *The Political Psychology of the Gulf War: Leaders, Publics, and the Process of Conflict*. Pittsburgh: University of Pittsburgh Press, pp. 29–48.

Weiss, Carol H. (1974). "What America's Leaders Read," *Public Opinion Quarterly* 38: 1–22.

Wilcox, Clyde, Joe Ferrara, and Dee Allsop (1991). "Before the Rally: The Dynamics of Attitudes Toward the Gulf Crisis Before the War," paper presented at the annual meeting of the American Political Science Association, Washington, DC.

Williams, W., Jr., and W. D. Semlak (1978). "Structural Effects of TV Coverage on Political Agendas," *Journal of Communication* 28: 114–19.

Winter, James P., and Chaim E. Eyal (1981). "Agenda Setting for the Civil Rights Issue," *Public Opinion Quarterly* 45: 376–83.

Wolfsfeld, Gadi (1983). "International Awareness, Information Processing, and Attitude Change: A Cross-Cultural Experimental Study," *Political Communication and Persuasion* 2: 127–46.

Zaller, John (1992). *The Nature and Origins of Mass Opinion.* New York: Cambridge University Press.

Index

203